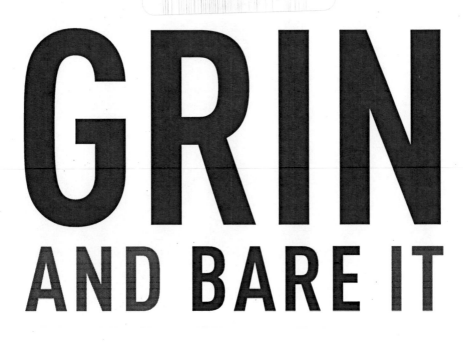

GRIN
AND BARE IT

GRIN
AND BARE IT

A Parent's Guide to Little Teeth

RANDY HAMILTON

Advantage®

Published by Advantage, Charleston, South Carolina.
Member of Advantage Media Group.

ADVANTAGE is a registered trademark and the Advantage colophon is a trademark of Advantage Media Group, Inc.

Printed in the United States of America.

ISBN: 978-159932-385-5
LCCN: 2013957204

This publication is designed to provide accurate and authoritative information in regard to the subject matter covered. It is sold with the understanding that the publisher is not engaged in rendering legal, accounting, or other professional services. If legal advice or other expert assistance is required, the services of a competent professional person should be sought.

Advantage Media Group is proud to be a part of the Tree Neutral® program. Tree Neutral offsets the number of trees consumed in the production and printing of this book by taking proactive steps such as planting trees in direct proportion to the number of trees used to print books. To learn more about Tree Neutral, please visit **www.treeneutral.com**. To learn more about Advantage's commitment to being a responsible steward of the environment, please visit **www.advantagefamily.com/green**

Advantage Media Group is a publisher of business, self-improvement, and professional development books and online learning. We help entrepreneurs, business leaders, and professionals share their Stories, Passion, and Knowledge to help others Learn & Grow. Do you have a manuscript or book idea that you would like us to consider for publishing? Please visit **advantagefamily.com** or call **1.866.775.1696**.

This book is dedicated to the many people in my life that have made this wonderful career possible. Rarely in life one gets an opportunity to spend time with kids all day, even at times be a kid yourself, and call it a career. Hopefully, there are even times where I help these children to realize the world is a better place because of them. I want to thank my parents who raised me to be the person I am today and always ingrained in me the confidence to accomplish anything. My wife who has stuck by my side from the beginning and never once complained about where we had to move or where we were living and struggled with me through all of our decisions. Finally, allow me to thank my iKids team. My vision for what iKids is all about would be impossible with out them. They all believe in the same vision and philosophy and I hope they all know how much they are appreciated.

Table of Contents

Introduction

AS A SPECIALIST in pediatric dentistry and a parent myself, I understand the desire parents have for honest, thoughtful answers to questions about their child's health care. We pore over books that outline our child's developmental progress, medical issues, and emotional health—but I'm surprised daily at the dearth of information even the best informed parents seem to have about their children's oral development and the important role that proper dental care plays in their overall health. It's not that they're not interested in the answers; it's simply that, outside of the dentist's office, they really have nowhere to turn for them. So many parents come in and ask me for answers to questions that should be common knowledge. They may have tried to do online research but still couldn't find reliable data. This book comes out of my desire to provide that vital information.

The whole topic of baby teeth deserves more attention than it gets. A lot of people say, "These teeth are going to fall out anyway, so why should I take care of them or worry about them?" Childhood is when you're establishing the habits for good oral health over your lifetime, habits that should be ingrained in the very beginning stages of life.

I start seeing patients at six months of age. Parents question why in the world I want to see infants when they don't even have any teeth, but it's not always about just the teeth. I'm concerned not only for their oral health care but for their overall health as well. When I'm seeing these infants, I'm talking to and educating the parents just as much as I am treating their children. I want to start seeing these patients early so that we can avoid any future problems by catching them before they become bigger issues, and I want to get the children used to the notion of the dentist. I urge parents to find somebody who specializes in pediatric dentistry.

Baby teeth are completely different than adult teeth. The enamel is thinner. The teeth obviously are not as mature. The anatomy of the teeth is different. The way that you treat a primary tooth is different from how you treat adult teeth.

Behavioral management is an art and a science. It's not something you can just pick up by being a mother or father. As I went into to my residency, I was already a father of four children, and it was amazing to me how little I knew about how to take a patient—a baby or a child—who was upset or traumatized and turn the situation around just through effective behavioral management. Now, I occasionally get a child who has been traumatized in the previous dentist's office and doesn't even want to sit down. By the time they leave, they're laughing; dental work is complete, and the child and parent had a great experience.

When you go to a dentist, you get a cleaning, exam, and radiographs. The most common question parents ask the dentist is, "Does my child have any cavities?" That's what most have come to expect from a dental visit. A dental visit should provide much more. The focus should be on the whole person and not just cavities. Of course, I look at that, but that's just one tiny aspect of what a comprehensive exam should be.

A comprehensive exam should cover growth and development of the child. Pathology on both soft and hard tissues should be examined. The occlusion or bite should be discussed as well as any evidence of crossbite, attrition, and erosion. That being said, hopefully, if anything is seen that could potentially stem from something wrong systemically, advice can be given to the parent to go to a physician who specializes in that specific area. Problems regarding the TMJ (temporormandibular joint), skeletal and tooth-related issues should also be covered.

Different types of x-rays may need to be taken in order to give the parents a more educated diagnosis on what is seen, such as malformations and missing teeth, and to allow us to observe overall development. Discussing what prevention methods would be beneficial is vital, in addition to discussing orthodontics, crowding, spacing issues, and periodontal issues.

Finally, trauma prevention, caries (cavities) risk and prevention, and diet should be discussed. There's a lot more to proper dental care than just checking for cavities.

Now, let's get down to the business of answering those questions—including some that may not have even occurred to you yet.

–RANDY W. HAMILTON, III DMD

Five Ways to Make Your Child's First Dental Visit an Experience You Want to Remember

1) SEEK OUT A PEDIATRIC DENTIST. Pediatric dental offices are set up specifically to ensure that children have a great experience. Pediatric dentists have multiple years of additional training in treating children's dental needs, their growth and development, the ability to observe pathology, special medical needs and syndromes, trauma, emergencies, and behavior management to make certain of a great experience. In addition, pediatric dentists are trained in different types of sedations for the timid, anxious, or extremely nervous child. We are in a new era of dentistry. There is no reason children should not have a fun, great experience at the dentist. Too many adults have grown up with a fear of the dentist that stems from too many bad experiences. A well-trained pediatric dentist can change that mindset. Remember, when a child has a great experience, the parents will have a great experience.

2) FIND A DENTIST THAT ALLOWS PARENTS INTO THE HYGIENE AND TREATMENT ROOMS. Too many dentist offices state they do not allow parents in treatment rooms because they want to build a relationship of trust or because they want kids to get used to the idea of being on their own. The dentist tells the parent that the child will do better without the parent there. In some instances, I agree. However, the majority of the time, I find that the parents stay out of the way and allow the dentist to do his job. I don't treat the child any differently based on whether or not Mom or Dad is in the room. In fact, I enjoy watching the parent see how well the child did and experience the visit with the child. I think some dentists are scared about what they will do in front of the parent if the child gets upset. Let's face it, anything new can be scary. Children always feel more comfortable if Mom or Dad can be there. We all feel more comfortable if we have someone else with us when we are trying something new. That doesn't apply solely to children; parents also feel more at ease because they can see what is going on and are able to be involved in the whole experience.

3) TAKE YOUR CHILD TO MEET THE DOCTOR AND STAFF AND TAKE A TOUR OF THE OFFICE BEFORE THE DENTAL VISIT. The day of the appointment holds a lot of anxiety; you can eliminate uncertainty on your child's part by letting her meet the dentist and staff in advance, which will lower the anxiety level. Just knowing what the office looks like will also remove some of the fear of the unknown.

4) GIVE POSITIVE REINFORCEMENT. I cannot count how may times I have met children who are terrified of the dentist because Mom and Dad told them they hate the dentist or said they are afraid of the dentist. I even have parents who tell their child they will get a big shot if they are not good. Wow! That would scare me. Instead, let your children know that the dentist is fun. Tell them the office is full of TVs, aquariums, video games, or flat screens on the ceiling with kids' movies playing (if it's true of your dentist's office, of course). Let your child know that this visit is special. Positive reinforcement goes a long way in helping your child have a great experience. If you want to go the extra mile, practice at home with your child, opening his mouth and pretending to count his teeth and then brushing his teeth as a hygienist might do.

5) BEGIN AND MAINTAIN GOOD ORAL HYGIENE HABITS AT HOME AND AT AN EARLY AGE. Brushing, flossing, and keeping your child familiar with good oral hygiene habits—along with a healthy diet—will also allow for a better visit to the dentist. When your children know they have been doing what they are supposed to do for their teeth at home, it makes for a very positive visit to the dentist. Contrary to popular belief, this is not the child's responsibility, but rather the parent's responsibility to ensure the child maintains good oral hygiene.

Chapter Two

When You're Expecting

IF YOU'RE EXPECTING, probably the last thing you're thinking about is your oral health. You're either excited or in shock when you find out you're pregnant; it's always one of the two (my wife and I have been through both of those: the planned-for and the surprise pregnancies). You're excited about picking out a name. You're excited about finding out if it's a boy or a girl. You're eager to see your doctor, first to make sure that you are pregnant, and then that the baby's okay. Oral health comes in last on your list, if it shows up at all.

DIET

When I talk with expectant mothers, I always want to start out with their diet. The mother's diet affects the health of the child, of course, and carbohydrates can also increase the risk of caries (cavities) for the mother. A lot of women fall into a snacking habit during their second and third trimesters, which means they're eating between meals without brushing. So if you're caving to your cravings for sugar, be sure to carry around a toothbrush. For convenience, you can even purchase a disposable toothbrush that already has toothpaste in it. In addition, chewing xylitol gum should become a habit. Xylitol is a sweetener that is as sweet as sucrose, but it's beneficial because it will actually reduce caries by a third and remineralize teeth. Look on the labels of different gums to see if they do indeed contain xylitol.

MORNING SICKNESS

Morning sickness and vomiting can also affect oral health. A majority of women experience some morning sickness, and the gastric acids of the stomach that are expelled in vomiting can erode a mother's teeth. When this happens, make sure to rinse your mouth out with water—or better yet—a fluoride rinse prior to brushing to counteract the acid.

GINGIVA HEALTH

From a periodontal perspective, hormone levels can affect the gingiva of the mother, which can lead to what's called "pregnancy gingivitis," when hormonal surges cause your gums or the gingiva to bleed, swell, and get painful. That's usually in the second trimester, and it will affect the front teeth more than the back teeth. Given this hormonally-caused gingivitis, the last thing we want is poor oral hygiene in mothers, because if you're not flossing or brushing your teeth, gingivitis may worsen.

What are the possible consequences if you don't take proper care of your teeth in this period? Poor plaque control can lead to gingivitis, causing increased bacteria; this inflammation can lead to periodontal issues, which in turn can cause bone loss and possibly mobile or loose teeth. Periodontitis can actually contribute to pre-term, low-birth-weight infants. The chance of complications for such a baby are increased, which can mean more time spent in the hospital for the infant.

Most of the time, you can control plaque just by brushing and flossing. But, as I've said, morning sickness can take a toll, too, if it causes vomiting, because gastric acid from the stomach can erode the back of your teeth. So, if you're dealing with morning sickness, take precautions and make sure that you rinse your mouth before your brush. Your first impulse, of course, is to grab your toothbrush, but don't; it's actually better just to rinse your mouth out really well afterward to get that acid off your teeth. You don't want to brush with toothpaste right after you've had that acid in your mouth because you would just be brushing that acid into the tooth, which would remove more enamel. It's better to rinse out, wait a little bit, and then go back and brush your teeth.

Pregnancy gingivitis occurs most often in the second trimester. Strictly speaking, we can't prevent it, but we need to keep it from getting worse by maintaining good home oral healthcare. That's your typical brushing—morning and night—and flossing.

Healthy eating habits play into oral health as well. Expectant moms tend to snack; you're just hungrier than usual, and if you're choosing wisely, that's not a bad thing. The key is that you want to stay away from food with lots of carbs. Your doctor will tell you, what you're eating is what you're giving to your baby, so you want to keep a healthy diet. As far as the potential impact on your oral health, the more carbohydrates you eat, the higher your risk of cavities becomes, and the higher the risk of pregnancy gingivitis as well.

19

Are there some things that might be better than others to snack on when you're not likely to brush your teeth immediately after snacking? Sure: fruits, vegetables, items that will not stick to your teeth. Raisins are not good, being high in sugar and very sticky. Maintaining a healthy diet is no different than when you're not pregnant. While you're pregnant, you have a tendency to rationalize that you're eating for two, but that's not necessarily the best way to approach it. There are a certain amount of calories that your physician wants you to eat per day, and it's not about eating for two. It's about maintaining a balanced diet and making it even richer in the nutrients the baby needs.

DENTIST VISITS

Women who are expecting are sometimes nervous about going to the dentist because it can involve x-rays and shots in your gums and so forth. Naturally, when you're expecting, your first impulse is to keep everything foreign away. But pregnant women need to keep to their schedule of annual visits, come in for a checkup, and come in for cleaning, because that's going to help with pregnancy gingivitis and help with maintaining good oral health. Our ultimate goal is to always protect the baby. With the technology that we have now in dentistry, it's not nearly as big a concern as it was even 10 years ago. We're also looking out for the comfort of the mother.

If you're expecting, and your teeth happen to need work but it's not an emergency, the most comfortable time for the dental work is between 14 and 20 weeks. You will be a lot more comfortable leaning back and getting treatment done at that point. In the first trimester, you definitely want to stay clear of nitrous oxide. In fact, I would suggest that you stay away from nitrous through your whole pregnancy. It's simply not worth risking your baby's health.

If an expectant mother has an emergency, no matter what point in their pregnancy, it's okay to go see the dentist and get out of pain. It is also okay to have a dental radiograph taken. The digital x-rays are phenomenal now in terms of the very limited exposure to radiation they create. How limited? The amount of exposure you get from one digital bitewing is about the same as you get walking from the door to your car outside. I'm speaking strictly about dental x-rays here, not about medical x-rays. That's a whole different ball game. The digital dental x-rays now usually don't even go past the other side of the face; still, I always want to use precautions when I use digital, or any type of x-ray. Be smart, use the lead apron and be conservative about the x-rays you take. Any time you get a dental x-ray, you should take care to have your thyroid shielded. That's just precautionary.

EMERGENCY CARE

Again, whether you're in your first, second, or third trimester, if there is an emergency, absolutely go into to see your dentist and don't be afraid to get an x-ray if you need it. If you're just going in for routine dental care or you know you have some cavities, you want to get taken care of, do it during the second trimester. During the first trimester, the risk of anything happening that might cause a miscarriage is just too great, and women who have been pregnant before will you tell you you're probably going to be miserable during the third trimester. You will probably have trouble sleeping at night and be uncomfortable sitting in one place for too long.

The second trimester is your safest and most comfortable period, so schedule your cleaning then. That will help to prevent any dental infections or periodontitis or any complications from occurring in the third trimester so you can just keep your mind on your baby.

Have a preventative plan with good oral hygiene. Make sure you are flossing, that you're rinsing out with some type of oral rinse. I've already discussed xylitol gum. Chew it multiple times a day. You can get it at any store now. In fact, if you check the labels, you will see that a lot of sugar-free gums have xylitol. I give it to children all the time.

Another concern is taking prescription drugs during pregnancy. Drugs fall into four categories: A, B, C, and D. Category A are drugs that have been studied in humans and have evidence supporting their safe use. Category B drugs show no evidence of risk to humans and are considered acceptable for use during pregnancy. Category C drugs are to be used with caution during pregnancy. Category D drugs are not intended for use during pregnancy. Your doctor will know what drugs fall into which group and will advise you accordingly.

If your doctor prescribes antibiotics during pregnancy, depending on when you're taking them, they can cause what's called hypo-calcification in your child's teeth. This appears as a yellowish or mottled enamel or even white areas on the teeth. These areas are weaker and more susceptible to cavities. The problems do not happen all the time; it all depends on when you're taking the antibiotics, the amount, and at the point at which the baby is born.

Your child's health comes first, so those spots may be something you really can't avoid. If you or your baby needs to be on those medications, you should take them. Those teeth are treatable once they come in.

To sum up: When you find out you're pregnant and you're scheduling all those doctor's visits you're going to need, make sure you also schedule your dentist visit. Do not neglect your oral health because your baby's health is tied to yours. If there are any nonemergency problems, you can wait until the second trimester to get them resolved. It would be nice to start your pregnancy with a nice clean, healthy mouth.

Chapter Three

Your Infant And Toddler, 0 To 24 Months

IDEALLY, YOUR BABY'S oral care begins at birth. In fact, while you're still in the hospital you can begin looking after your baby's oral health. After you give the bottle to or nurse the baby, go ahead and wipe his gums. This gets the baby used to having something in his mouth, and begins the process of preventative oral care. You can use a clean washcloth or any damp, clean cloth; it doesn't matter what it is as long as it's clean.

When you're cleaning your infant's mouth, you're going to go over the whole mouth. You're going to go around the cheeks, the ridges where the teeth come in, everywhere that the milk has been, and you're going to wipe the tongue as well. Then as those first teeth start to come in around six months, go ahead and pull out a toothbrush. It needs to be a really soft toothbrush, a smaller toothbrush than an adult size. You don't need to use toothpaste at this time. You're just trying to get off the little bit of the film left from the milk, rice cereal or whatever the baby is eating.

STAYING STERILE

There are three things needed to cause cavities: sugar, bacteria, and teeth. When a baby is first born, the mouth is sterile. The longer we keep it sterile, the better we will be. We want to do all we can to avoid transmitting the bacteria from your mouth, from another baby's mouth, or from grandparents' mouth to the infant's mouth. The way infants most commonly get this bacteria is through this kind of transmission, whether it comes from parents cleaning the pacifier with their mouth and then giving it back to the baby, or, when they're spoon-feeding the baby, taking the spoon and touching it to their tongue to test how hot the food is before putting it into the baby's mouth. Even something as simple as Grandma and Grandpa wanting to smooch on their little grandbaby by kissing her on the mouth transfers bacteria from their mouth into the babys. All of a sudden this baby goes from having a sterile mouth to one with potentially cavity-causing bacteria. The longer you can avoid getting that bacteria into your baby's mouth, the longer it is before we have to worry about cavities.

We call it horizontal transmission or vertical transmission. Vertical transmission is right from the mouth of a parent, from Mom's or Dad's mouth to the baby's mouth. Horizontal transmission comes from other people or grandparents. In the exam room, I counsel parents to look out for this kind of transmission, to try to avoid kissing the baby on or around the mouth, although I know it's hard, because those cheeks are big and those babies are cute.

EARLY TEETH

Occasionally, a baby is actually born with a tooth, which is called a natal tooth. A neo-natal tooth is one that comes in shortly thereafter. These unexpected teeth can scare a parent. Many times the parent has no idea what is going on, or are spooked that the baby has a tooth, but it's nothing to be frightened by. When these early teeth come in, there are a couple of things that we can do with it, depending on the circumstances. If it is solidly in place, we will leave it there because it is that baby's primary tooth. He won't get another to replace it. On the other hand, if the tooth is mobile (loose), our biggest concern is that it will fall out on its own and the baby will inhale it and stop breathing. If the tooth is mobile, I will go ahead and extract it. It's a very simple procedure. I use very minimal anesthesia, and the baby can sit on Mom or Dad's lap. It takes two seconds to remove the tooth. Unfortunately, another baby tooth will not grow into that spot, but we are protecting your baby from potentially aspirating a tooth and that's more important.

Typically, a baby gets her first teeth about six months of age, and the first two teeth to appear are normally the lower front teeth. You'll find a tooth eruption chart at the end of the book for quick reference. This is merely meant as a guide, not law. It's okay if your child isn't following the norm. "Typical" is the important word here; parents will come in worried because their child is seven or eight months old, and they don't have any teeth. But it's nothing to worry about.

When we do those averages, it's the pediatric dentists and the orthodontists who usually determine when those teeth are coming in. We just give it an average, but of course every child is different. There are children that may have every single one of their teeth by the time they are 10 or 12 months old. There are other children who may be two and a half years old and not have all of their teeth yet. It's just an average, so there's no real reason to be concerned if your child is a little late hitting that benchmark. Eventually, those teeth will come in.

FIRST VISIT TO DENTIST

The emergence of your child's first tooth is a good time for the first visit to the dentist. A lot of new mothers wonder why I ask them to bring their infants in to see the dentist this early. The thinking on this first visit has changed significantly in the last 10 to 20 years, although even today some pediatricians may say the child's first dental visit doesn't need to be until age three. Please don't wait until three. We need to get these children in no later than their first birthdays, not only for the children but also for the parent's education as well. Pediatric dentists know it is important to establish your child's dental home early just as it is the medical home. We are working on educating pediatricians on this as well. We want to create a comfortable place where parents feel confident in bringing their children. And we want to start building a trusting relationship with your children, so that they grow up feeling comfortable with the dentist.

At that initial visit, the child sits in your lap for what's called a "lap exam." I typically begin by going over your baby's medical and family history. It's important that I know whether your child was born full term and whether he had any pertinent medical issues when he was born. If he was born pre-term, then there's a possibility that the child was on a respirator. This is important information for any future visits in case I have to use sedation or perform any work on your child. More importantly, I want to have this information in our medical history in case any type of emergency does happen.

At that first visit, I also discuss trauma. I go over when teeth will be coming in and what to expect. I also want to know family history and find out whether Mom and Dad have had cavities and how their oral hygiene is. This helps us determine the caries risk for the baby and consider possible future treatment and/or preventative treatment.

The way a lap exam works is that Mom will be sitting down, the baby will be sitting down in her lap as if she is giving Mom a hug, and Mom will lean the baby back into the doctor's lap. If the baby has teeth, I will go over every single tooth, and make sure that there's no pathology on the teeth such as cavities. I'll be looking at the cheeks, under the tongue, and around the lips, to make sure there's no pathology there. I'll look at both the hard and the soft palate and make sure those are fully formed. Then I go in and discuss proper ways to care for the mouth and the teeth. If there are no teeth in place yet, I explain the process of wiping the gums. If there are teeth, I show you how to get started using a toothbrush on your baby's teeth. Depending on the child, a discussion should take place regarding the child's development including crawling, walking, speaking, and social behavior.

TOOTHBRUSHES, TOOTHPASTE, FLOSS, AND SEALANTS

I also talk about what type of toothpaste to use. Typically I don't advise parents to start using fluoride toothpaste until most of the anteriors are in or the first molars begin to come in. At that point, you can use just a little smear; not even a pea-size amount of toothpaste. Remember, their mouths are smaller, and they have fewer teeth. A little bit of toothpaste goes a long way.

When you do start using fluoride toothpaste, it's important that you get those fluoride ions absorbed into the teeth. The latest literature shows that the actual topical application is the best way to get fluoride into the teeth, so having the fluoride on the teeth rather than introducing it systemically does a much better job. When your child is around two to three years, you can use just a pea-sized portion of toothpaste. This way the child can swallow the toothpaste and it will not hurt them. That's the parents' main concern; "If he swallows toothpaste, my child can't spit." That's okay, as long as you use a small amount, he can swallow it and it will not affect him.

I tell parents I do not want their children to rinse their mouths out after brushing. Once they learn to spit, that's great; they can spit the toothpaste out and can go on their way. But the whole benefit of fluoride toothpaste is to get these fluoride ions absorbed in the teeth and rinsing negates that. Fluoride changes the whole structure of the tooth and makes the tooth harder and less susceptible to cavities. That's our goal. Rinsing your mouth after brushing rinses all the fluoride off. It takes about 20 or 30 minutes for the fluoride to be absorbed into the teeth after the teeth are brushed. Rinsing out your mouth completely goes against what we're trying to do. Spit and go on your way.

Around age 2, your child should have her full complement of teeth or close to it. This is the time that a scary word arises for parents: "floss." The dental profession has done a tremendous job in making brushing fun. Toothbrushes light up, vibrate, even sing. However, we have done a lousy job in making flossing fun. One company has turned the tide. If you want your children to *ask* to floss their teeth, get them Gum Chucks. It is the newest innovation in flossing and is fun for children and adults alike.

Your pediatric dentist should also take this opportunity to discuss other preventative strategies. Along with the use of fluoride toothpaste, when the child is old enough to work with, I recommend putting sealants on the molars that need them. For those who do not know, sealants are protective coatings that are placed in the grooves and fissures of molars and premolars. The sealants fill in these pits and fissures so the toothbrush may cleanse the entire surface of the tooth without missing those deeper areas. This move is preventative because bacteria are small enough to sneak down in those crevices in teeth where the brush bristles are too large to reach. If the patient lives in an area where the water is not fluoridated, this would be the time to discuss using fluoride supplements, in addition to fluoride toothpaste, depending on the caries risk.

BOTTLES, CUPS, AND HEALTHY TEETH

Most parents have heard the phrase "baby bottle tooth decay." Unfortunately, it still exists. You should aim to get your baby off the bottle by 12 months or to stop nursing by 18 months. Even more importantly than getting your baby off the bottle by the age of 12 months, I want to encourage you not to send your baby to bed with a bottle. As a parent myself, I know this is easier said than done. For those of us who have kids, I know all parents have come to that night where they've had a long day, the baby's fussing, and it's easier to just give him a bottle and put him in his crib or bed, where he's happy. You have quiet for once and can have that precious little span of alone time. We've all been there. That said, it's really important that we try not to fall into that habit. What happens is the baby has a sucking reflex, so he's going to be sucking but a lot of times won't swallow the milk. It will just pool up around his front teeth. If this continues to occur, those teeth will begin to decay and what we normally think of as a slow process will happen rather quickly. The same occurs with nursing.

The ideal way to handle the bedtime feeding is to hold your baby, give her the bottle to fill her tummy up, wipe her mouth or brush her teeth, then put her to bed. Again, I know it's easier said than done—but it's very important to make that your routine. Once those teeth start coming in, we really have to watch what we do and especially avoid putting the baby to bed with the bottle.

PACIFIERS

Another topic I discuss in the lap exam are habits like sucking, not only pacifiers but also thumbs and fingers. Pacifiers are fine in the beginning stages of life if that's what you want to use to comfort your baby, but you need to make sure that you get rid of the pacifiers by the time your child turns two. It's crucial, because what we see with pacifiers most often is that it causes a crossbite. With a normal bite, when your teeth are closed, the top teeth overlap the bottom teeth. It's just the opposite with a crossbite; the bottom teeth overlap the top teeth. That's only corrected with a palatal expander or braces, and that can't happen until your child is six to ten years old. They will have to live with this crossbite once it's formed until we can correct it, so it's much easier if we avoid the crossbite altogether.

Habits can be hard to break for anyone and stopping the pacifier once it's become a habit isn't easy, but I have a couple of tricks to help you out. One is to cut the tip off of the pacifier and then hand it back to your baby. Once the tip is cut off, your child cannot get that sucking sensation in their mouth, so a baby will just throw the pacifier away. If your child is already two or three years old, I suggest that you get a helium balloon, tie the pacifier onto that balloon, then walk outside with your child and say it's time for the pacifier to go to another baby. Then let the child release the balloon. That way, they can watch their pacifier float away to some other baby somewhere, and it feels more like a minor rite of passage than a loss. Another alternative is to discontinue it at once rather than weaning off of it. It's going to be hard for about a week; however, the child will forget about the pacifier.

I hear many parents stating they have tried everything to break their child of the pacifier habit, including coating it with spicy sauce. I do not advise putting any type of pepper or hot sauce on the end of the pacifier. To me, that's traumatizing your baby, and there's no reason to do that.

EATING AND DRINKING

Another item I discuss during the lap exam is your baby's diet. Typically, an infant is drinking either breast milk or formula and some water, and perhaps eating rice cereal. That's all fine, but a buzzword for me is "juice." As soon as I hear "juice," I let the parent know to be cautious with juice as a food for the baby. Juice does not have much nutritional value. Still, we need to be realistic. A child could live off milk and water alone the rest of their life, but that doesn't make life much fun. I don't have a problem with giving a child juice every once in a while, but you should limit it to snack and meal times so they drink the juice at one sitting. Allowing your child to walk around with a bottle full of juice is a very bad idea, since juice is so high in sugar. It is the same for sugary drinks such as soda, Kool-aid, etc. Remember, it's the constant exposure to the sugar that causes cavities.

If your child is at 12 months of age, I want you to switch the child off the bottle. Here's a good technique: if your child prefers milk to water, go ahead and switch him to a sippy cup. At nighttime, or anytime when your child requests a bottle, have the sippy cup and the bottle sitting there in front of him. Put milk in the sippy cup, put water in the bottle, and let him choose. The child will usually choose the milk, and you start to wean him off the bottle then and there. You can also do it cold turkey. It makes for about a good long week of crying, but your baby will eventually forget about the bottle, and then you move on. Any time you give your baby a bottle of anything other than water, as I said before, you should go in and wipe off the baby's mouth.

Once your children start having rice cereal or when they start eating purees of your table food, make sure that what you're giving them is healthy. Limit sugary snacks to once or twice a day. When I say sugary snacks, I not only mean solid foods, but drinks too, like juice or chocolate milk. If you're going to offer juice and chocolate milk, again, you should do it at snack and meal time only. Do not put it in their sippy cups and allow them to walk around and consistently soak their teeth. What causes cavities most is the length of time that the sugar sits on teeth. If sugary drinks are consumed in one sitting, the saliva actually has time to rinse off the teeth and helps with the prevention of cavities. If your children are consistently coating their teeth with the juice they have in their sippy cup, and they go back every five minutes because the juice is sitting on the table for them to drink, their saliva does not have time to rinse their teeth off.

With snacks, it's the same advice. Refrain from always giving your kids chocolate chip cookies, M&Ms, gummy bears, gummy worms, or other sugary snacks. Try to get the child into the habit of eating healthy snacks. If you can do that early on, that's what the child will want. If you get your child in the habit of eating sugary things early on, then your child is going to want sugary things. You're in the power position at this point in your children's lives in terms of what they eat, and you can do them a big favor by helping them to develop good eating habits for life.

KEEPING LITTLE MOUTHS SAFE

At around eight months to 12 months of age, something to consider is whether your child is mobile and how mobile. Can you lay him in the middle of the blanket, walk out of the room, and find him still on the blanket when you come back? Or are you at that stage where you lay your child in the middle of the blanket, walk out of the room, come back and discover that he's missing? Parents laugh at that, but it's true. If you have kids yourself, you know exactly what I'm talking about—that panicky feeling parents know all too well.

Children are teething by the time that they're crawling, and anything they can get in their mouths, they will. Anything they can wrap in their hands is that much easier to put in their mouths. They like little, hard, plastic things that feel good to their aching gums and make that sensitivity go away. Electric cords are at the top of the popularity chart. It's extremely important that when your children become mobile, you find a way to hide electric cords so they can't get to them, because they will wrap their little hands around the cord and it goes right into their mouth. Cords are fun to chew on because they're little and they're hard, so the kids just gnaw and gnaw. If there's a break in the electric cord, or if your baby's little sharp teeth get through the cord, then you have a very serious problem on your hands. It's called electric burn. This electric burn will stay with them for the rest of their lives and is a difficult thing to treat. I can tell you I have seen this, and it's a sad sight. There are various kinds of cord covers available, just as there are covers sold for outlets and power strips. Use them. You can't be too vigilant when it comes to childproofing your house because there is no end to the things babies will find and swallow or aspirate. Too many infants and toddlers wind up in the ER after swallowing items their caretakers overlooked. Do not forget to unplug your phone cords after charging. These cords fit well into small hands and could easily cause an electric burn.

DEALING WITH TEETHING

Another topic I talk about in this lap exam, especially the first appointment, is teething. I discuss how your baby's teeth will start to come in at five or six months and what you can do to ease your child's teething pain. The first thing I recommend is Children's

Tylenol or Children's Motrin. For one thing, this allows the child to be able to sleep through the night. If the child gets a better night's rest, it's going to be not only easier for the child but also for you the next day. Teething tablets also work well. A lot of my parents use teething tablets and like them. I don't recommend teething gels very often because when you put teething gel in one spot it tends to travel around the mouth via the saliva and all of a sudden your baby's whole mouth is numb. That's not a fun feeling for anyone. Chewing brings your child relief, especially if the chew toy is cold, so put it in the freezer.

How do you know when your child is teething? Some children will start salivating more. Some children will start putting their fingers in their mouths and chewing on their fingers. Anything else they can get hold of will start going in their mouths: toys, blankets, etc. Some children will run a slight fever. This fact is important: typically, fever caused by teething will usually not go above 100.3 degrees. That's the magic number. If your baby's fever is over 100.3, then you should consider that this might be a sinus infection or ear infection and go see your baby's physician.

PREPARING FOR TRAUMA

Once children are mobile, we always hope for the best, but we want to be prepared for the worst because trauma can be an issue. By the time children are a year old, they're trying to walk or trying to lift themselves up. Their chins or their mouths can hit tables, or they can fall and hit their faces on the floor, and you want to be prepared for that. Once that happens—because it will—before you panic, assess the situation. Get your child, get a wet rag, wipe away the blood, and then look to see where the blood is coming from. If your child has a fractured tooth or has knocked out a tooth, you need to try to find the tooth and make sure the baby didn't swallow it. Call your pediatric dentist immediately. Many times, unless you take your baby to a children's hospital, an ER physician will not know what to do in this situation, so you need to find a pediatric dentist that is on call. Be sure to have your pediatric dentist's number programmed in your phone so you will not have to search for it in an emergency.

Luckily, most of the time, a fall will only cause a minor laceration in your child's mouth. Little lacerations to the mouth will typically heal themselves, and you don't need to worry about little bumps and bruises. Your baby has a little attachment, called the frenum, that I talk to parents about in a lap exam. The frenum is the flap of tissue that attaches the gum to the lip. This tears very easily, and when it tears, it bleeds a lot. That is a very common occurrence when infants fall. When that happens, do not panic. Get a wet rag and put pressure on the wound for about 10 minutes. It will stop bleeding, and nothing else needs to be done about it. A parent's first instinct when they see all the blood from a frenum tear is to head to the ER, but the tear will heal fine on its own.

Very often I have parents come in and tell me, "My child won't let me brush his teeth." Most young children do not want someone else's hands in their mouth brushing their teeth for them, and if you have not started doing this for your children early, it's harder to accustom them to it later. But you need to use tough love in this situation, because having a child cry for about two to three minutes while you're brushing her teeth is so much better than allowing her to get cavities. If she does, then we have to go in and risk a possible sedation in order to fix her teeth. You can't fall back on the excuse that, "My child will not let me brush her teeth." We're the parents, and we know what's best for our children, even when they don't like it.

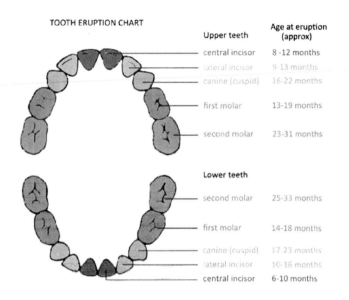

American Academy of Pediatric Dentistry
Pediatric Dentistry-Reference Manual

Chapter Four

Your Child From Ages Two To Six

THE KEY TO THIS PERIOD of your child's development from a dentist's point of view is continuing the development of good habits, both for the children and the parents. By age 2, your child starts to feel more independent (my wife and I often discuss whether it's actually the Terrible Twos or the Terrible Threes). This is the time to start implementing floss in addition to brushing, since all the teeth have come in at this age. "Floss" can be a frightening word for a lot of parents. Brushing twice a day is difficult enough, they feel, and now I'm asking them to start implementing floss? I understand. Automatically starting to floss seven days a week is ideal. However, let's be realistic. I suggest you start out at two or three days a week in the beginning, in order to get both you and your child used to this new habit—and a habit is what it needs to become.

HOW TO BRUSH

Many parents ask me how they can brush and floss their child's teeth well at this age. Basically, every parent needs to find out which techniques to use, based on your own child's personality and needs. There are several techniques you can use. You can use distraction, with something as simple as giving a child a book to look at, turning on her favorite show, or letting her hold a stuffed animal. You can do what I call, "Tell, Show, Do." Tell the child what you're going to do, show your child how you brush your own teeth, and then go and brush hers. You can turn it in to a game.

Parents will come back and say, "We've tried all that, and it doesn't work." Folks, that's where the tough love comes into play. Fortunately, parents do know best and forcing your child to brush his teeth is, at times, necessary. I've heard moms say regarding a two-year-old child, "He just will not let me brush his teeth." I tell the parent that as long as you are larger, he should not have a choice. When Mom says, "I just can't hold him down and I don't want to turn this into an issue," my response is that it's your choice—but it seems to me that it shows more love to actually hold him down and brush his teeth than the alternative, which is allowing your child to get a cavity and then the child having to make an extra trip to the dentist's office to get anesthetics or, at that age, probably sedation, in order to fill it.

Unfortunately, the option to that dentist trip is leaving the cavity to get larger and spread, which it will,[9] until multiple teeth have cavities. Then, we'll have to use an antibiotic to take care of the infection, and we'll have to extract the infected teeth because you cannot save an infected primary tooth like you can an adult tooth. Additionally, once the baby tooth is infected, it also puts the permanent teeth at risk for damage—and all of this because you were not willing to hold a child a little bit while you brushed her teeth? Clearly, we need to get our priorities straight here.

GOING SOLO

Parents will also come in and say, "When can they brush for themselves?" My hygienist says they're ready to brush their own teeth when they can tie their shoe and it stays tied all day (yes, I know what you're thinking—there are a lot of adults who shouldn't be brushing their own teeth either!) Children will not have the dexterity to brush their own teeth for a while. However, I want your child to have that sense of accomplishment and independence, so I do recommend that parents let them try to brush on their own, then follow up and go over their brushing job, while letting them know what a good job they did. Children should not begin to brush their own teeth until age nine or 10, and parents should still check to be sure they're doing it correctly.

When I was little, Mom or Dad would come in and check to see if my toothbrush was wet. Well, I knew how to get around that—just stick the toothbrush under the faucet and go to bed. What I recommend to make sure your child has actually brushed (and you don't have to do it every time because some parents might think it's a little gross) is to make sure your hands are clean, then take your fingernail and actually scrape your child's front tooth to see if you can scrape any plaque off. If you do find plaque, then your child needs to understand that Mom or Dad will be brushing for them for the next two or three days. When you don't scrape any plaque off, then they can continue brushing on their own.

Another way to show your child what spots he's missing while brushing is with a special colored mouth rinse that's available. After children brush their teeth, they can rinse or swish this around their mouth, then spit it out, and it will show blue or green all around the areas of the tooth that they've missed. I do recommend trying that, because it is a wonderful way to help older children figure out which parts of their teeth they're missing with their brushing routine.

THE RIGHT KIND OF TOOTHBRUSH

Parents often ask me what type of toothbrush they should be using, and my answer is always, "Whatever the child *will* use." Toothbrushes can be age-specific. If your child wants a cartoon character toothbrush and that's what it takes to motivate the brushing, get one. Parents will also ask, "Is a mechanical toothbrush any better than a manual toothbrush?" The answer is not necessarily. If you're using a manual toothbrush, as long as you're using it correctly, it can be as effective as a mechanical toothbrush. A lot of children prefer mechanical toothbrushes, because they make brushing more fun. It doesn't matter what type of toothbrush as long as they're using it correctly, and if a mechanical toothbrush helps with that, there's nothing wrong with letting them use it. In addition, make sure the brush has soft bristles.

FUN WITH FLOSSING

Flossing can be made to be more exciting as well. Make it a game. Have siblings race. Have children time themselves to break their previous record. There are flossers with different characters as well as the newest flossing utensils called Gum Chucks. They look like nunchucks and keep your fingers out of your mouth. And even more fun, after you're finished flossing with Gum Chucks, you press two buttons and the floss goes flying in the air. My kids love the Gum Chucks, and it has given them something to actually look forward to when they floss.

Parents also want to know what type of toothpaste the child should be using. It really doesn't matter, as long as it does have fluoride in it. Some parents will say, "My children don't like that minty taste." The good news is there are lots of toothpastes out there that don't have the minty taste, and as long as they have fluoride, they're just fine. That said, I would recommend staying away from whitening toothpaste because it's too abrasive for little teeth. As to the amount the child should use, stay with a pea-sized portion or smaller in the toddler years since they still may not be spitting.

Here's an interesting and potentially life-saving little fact. It takes about seven or eight milligrams of fluoride per kilogram of the child's weight in order to make a child sick. If they get that amount when you're not looking, you make them drink a glass of milk, and monitor them. You need to know the weight of your child and then do that math to find out "What is the amount that can actually hurt my child?" As long as you stick to the pea-sized portion, you're not going to get anywhere close to that amount.

TRIPS TO THE DENTIST WITH A TODDLER

What should you expect when you take your two- or three-year-old child to the dentist? When your child is age two, your dentist is still probably going to be a doing a lap exam. We're going to be discussing diet, especially at the toddler age, because this is when your children are making more of their food choices on their own and they are wanting to snack more. Again, I'll go through and check every single tooth, and I want to make sure that the child is getting good oral hygiene and brushing morning and night. I'll talk about implementing flossing with the parents. Then I'll do what's called a toothbrush prophy, which is a gentle cleaning with a toothbrush to remove plaque from your child's teeth and gums. I will probably not take x-rays of a two-year-old unless I see something that warrants it. Just as I did in examining the younger child, I'll check around for any visible pathology.

The child will get a fluoride treatment, and the fluoride that I prefer to give to children is a varnish. The reason for that is that the varnish actually absorbs better, sticks to the teeth longer, and the child does not have to wait 30 minutes to eat or drink—which is a big plus when you're a child. That is the one thing that I remember I hated when I went to the dentist as a kid: having to wait 30 minutes in addition to having to keep that stuff in your mouth for two whole minutes and swish. I never knew that my facial muscles could be sore until I had to do that.

TALKING ABOUT SNACKING

In this exam, I'm going to discuss sugar intake. As parents, we want to limit our kids' sugar intake, not only for their oral health but because too much sugar can cause other health issues as well. A big dose of sugar can cause a hyperactive period followed by a "crash"; taking in too much sugar on a regular basis can cause weight gain and keeps your body from being as healthy as it can be. Can you take away sugar completely from your children? Well, no. They're children, and we need to be realistic given the society in which we live. I don't have any problem with the occasional candy bar but, just as with anything else, you want to be wise about it. Limit your child's sugary snacks to one or two a day.

All-day snacking has become dangerously ingrained in our parenting practices. Who hasn't seen kids toting those little plastic snack containers full of dry cereal or miniature snack crackers? We tend to think of those as harmless snacks, but those snack crackers and cereal stick to your child's teeth—and that allows the bacteria in their mouths to have a field day. Basically it's a bacteria buffet all day long, and that's really destructive to those teeth. When you give your child a snack like that, you should be brushing their teeth after that snack—not giving them little totes to carry the snacks around with them. Rather than dry cereal or snack crackers, I'd like see parents giving their kids healthy snacks like carrots or fruits. Dice up strawberries, or grab a handful of blueberries and put those in their little containers. Your saliva can wash those off your teeth a lot easier than Goldfish or Cheez-its.

Let's also talk about liquids. You want to limit your child's sugary drinks to snack or mealtime. Remember, as we've talked about before, it's the consistency with which the sugar stays on the teeth that causes cavities. If you're going to give your child chocolate milk or the occasional soda, do it at snack and meal times so she will drink it all at once and then be done with it. If you're going to give a child a sippy cup or a little thermos to walk around with all day, it needs to contain water. She needs to get into the habit of drinking water when she's thirsty, so limit sugary drinks to snack and meal times and stick with water during the rest of the day.

At age two the child should be off the bottle and by now should also be through with the pacifier. At this visit, I'll look at the cavity risks again and look at whether your child has had any previous decay or missing teeth, or if your child is considered to have what's called early childhood caries, which is a specific diagnosis to that age group.

SPECIAL MEDICAL NEEDS CHILDREN

If your child has special medical needs, I'm going to treat him just as we do any other. I want to get a good cleaning done and check every single tooth. That way I can form a diagnosis and treatment plan. I'll talk more about working with special medical needs children in a later chapter, but I'd like to say here, as a parent, that I want you to know your special medical needs child is the same as any other child in my dental office. What I mean by this is that their needs in terms of treatment are just like everyone else's in my waiting room, and that is a marvelous feeling to have for your child and for you as a parent.

BREAKING BAD HABITS

Now, let's talk about some of those habits your child may have that can affect the teeth and the mouth shape. Because the mouth is continuing to develop, habits like reliance on the pacifier or thumb- or finger sucking can be detrimental. This is the age at which we want to get rid of these habits. Let's talk the about pacifier first. While using a pacifier is perfectly all right for an infant, by the time your child turns two, it can begin to do some real damage. It can actually cause the space between the canines or the inter-canine distance to narrow, which is a bad thing. It can cause the palate to be high. It can cause an open bite in the front teeth. It can cause a crossbite on the back teeth, which is very difficult to correct. For those who don't know what a crossbite is; your top teeth normally overlap your bottom teeth by a couple of millimeters, but with a crossbite, the bottom teeth will overlap the top teeth. When this happens, the midline of your front teeth will no longer be aligned.

After age two, the damage will continue to get worse with the pacifier. Parents will tell me, "I bought that orthodontic pacifier," they found at the store; however, that's not going to help either. It will still do damage.

Thumb sucking is next in line in terms of damage. The thumb will also cause a high palate and will cause a flare of the front teeth just like the pacifier will. When it comes to breaking the pacifier habit, you can throw a pacifier away. You can't just throw a thumb away, so thumb sucking can be a more difficult habit to break.

How do we break children of these habits? I talked earlier about cutting off the tip of the pacifier, which will cause the child to lose the sucking sensation and reject it; alternately, you can make a rite of passage out of it with your child, tying the pacifier to a balloon to send to a baby who needs it. Reassure the child that she is growing up and doesn't really need it any more.

To help break the thumb-sucking habit, there is a product called Mavala that works wonders. I heard about this product from a colleague of mine and couldn't believe I had not been using it before. In fact, I've cured my own three older children of biting their fingernails with it. It's not spicy; it's not hot; and it will not hurt your child—but it just tastes awful. It looks like a clear finger-nail polish, and it's designed specifically for breaking habits such as fingernail biting or thumb sucking. You paint it on your child's thumb or fingernail and once he's tasted it, he will not want to place his thumb in his mouth any more. It works wonderfully.

If nighttime is the only time that thumb sucking is a problem, I recommend getting long-sleeve pajamas and sewing a sock on the end of the sleeve. That will keep the thumb out of your child's mouth throughout the night. However, do not take the shortcut; I've had more than one dad tell me that they could not believe their child bit through duct tape.

Do no forget about positive reinforcement, and a little bribery. In the beginning, if your child has gone one full day without putting her thumb in her mouth, then she gets to go to the dollar store or something along those lines, and pick out a prize. Extend it two days, then three days, then five days, with each milestone earning your child some kind of small prize. Once you get up to that 30-day mark, you're in pretty good shape. Your child is not going to go back to that habit.

Parents ask me, "Can you just put in an appliance?" I prefer the appliance be used as a last resort. Once they get to be around age six or seven, that's when I will run interference if I need to.

A GRINDING PROBLEM

Have you ever been awakened from a deep sleep by a horrible sound that you could not at first identify? You wake up and follow the sound that appears to be coming from one part of the house but also sounds like it might be two skeletons fighting on your roof. You track the noise to your child's room and realize the ferocious sound is coming from your child's mouth. Grinding is very normal in children at this age. Between the ages of two to six, it actually does get worse, and louder and louder. In most instances, it does not do any damage to the primary teeth. We don't really know the true cause of it. Children are figuring out all these new teeth in their mouths and how they sound and how they feel. Some may think that these children may have had a pacifier before and now that they're through with the pacifier, they're just kind of biting down on their own teeth. But all of my children have ground their teeth, and none of them used a pacifier, so I don't think that's the cause.

Another reason might be children are just trying to find their occlusion (or how the teeth are to sit against one another). Once their permanent teeth start to come in, which begins with their six-year molars, their occlusion tends to shift a little bit and change. The majority of the time children quit grinding their teeth at that point. It's funny; my six-year-old has now stopped grinding her teeth but for the last two to three years, she would wake us up at night with the noise.

Lip biting is a problem sometimes for this age group, although I see it more often in a slightly older patient. The key to breaking this habit is positive reinforcement, and helping the child to remember. If the child is a little older, like 8 to 10 years old, you can go to the store and get them a little sports mouth guard they can put in at night and that will keep them from biting their lip as well as grinding. I had a 10-year-old patient who almost bit through her own lip. Whether it's merely a habit or related to anxiety or stress varies from child to child.

CAVITIES IN TODDLERS

When we find cavities in your two-year-old's teeth, they need to be treated. A lot of parents ask, "These teeth are baby teeth and are going to fall out anyway. Why do they need to be filled?" There are various reasons. Baby teeth serve two important purposes; one is to assist them in their speech, and the other is to guide their permanent teeth in. Those baby teeth are acting as natural space maintainers. Once a tooth gets a cavity, if it's in between the teeth, that cavity's going to start eating away at that tooth and the teeth behind are going to start shifting forward to fill in the space. Your child is going to start losing space. Permanent teeth can be blocked out from erupting, or coming in properly.

Cavities in baby teeth will progress faster than they do in adult teeth, just because of the anatomy of the baby teeth: the enamel is thinner, and the pulp chambers are larger in baby teeth. So once a cavity starts forming, it spreads pretty quickly and it can get into the nerve. Once it gets into the nerve, it can cause an infection, and that infection can go down and damage the permanent tooth and cause the child pain. That is why we need to take care of cavities even when they are in baby teeth.

Children won't lose these first molars until they're 9 or 10 years old, usually. They won't lose their second molars until they're anywhere from 11 to 12 years old. If a child does lose a tooth, and if the permanent tooth is not going to be coming in soon, we do need to replace that baby tooth with a space maintainer to protect that space. Otherwise, if one of those permanent teeth gets blocked out, we're in a lot of trouble.

NON-TRAUMA CARE

A pediatric dentist's job is not only to manage the oral care of children—from usually zero to 18—but it's also to make sure these children have a good experience and do not become traumatized. How many adults do you know who hate to go to the dentist and put off care they should be getting to avoid the dentist's chair, even when they know better? Most often this behavior stems from unpleasant, uncomfortable, or frightening experiences they had when they were young.

A specialist's job is to turn that around. The training we have in behavior management allows us to go in and treat these children without upsetting them, whether they are awake or asleep, and exceeds the training you commonly find in general and family dentists. Can a lot of children go to a family dentist and be fine? Absolutely. Many family dentists are great with children. However, one bad experience is all it takes. Once that happens, the specialist has to undo the damage and work through the fear the child already has. I have to bring them back to square one, whereas if they had been at the specialist's office in the first place it wouldn't have been necessary.

No parent wants to see their child suffering or in pain. I've seen too many children go to the dental offices where they are held down and they're not sedated while the work is being done. The parent isn't allowed in the room with them, so they don't even know what's going on or why their child is crying. "Why do you do that to children?" I asked one of my colleagues who owns several general dental offices where they typically see a lot of kids. He shrugged it off. "Oh, kids are resilient. They'll scream and cry for about an hour, but they'll bounce right back." I personally just think that is wrong. I would not want my child to have to go through that, and I don't want anyone else's child to have to go through that.

As a specialist, if a child can't handle treatment under regular behavior management, I can try nitrous. If nitrous with behavior management doesn't work, then I have the tools to go in and do oral sedation. If the oral sedation doesn't work, then I have the training to do IV sedation. If IV sedation doesn't work, then we have the capacity to take the child into the hospital or the operating room and put them under general anesthesia. That way this child can have a great experience, get all the teeth done at the same time, and doesn't have that fear of coming to the dentist.

I tell my parents, "Look, the reason that we offer this is so that when you tell your child that you're taking her to see Dr. Hamilton, I want the child to start jumping up and down and run to the car. I don't want the child to run and hide in the corner."

Fear comes from having a bad experience or watching others have bad experiences. Many times parents serve as their child's security blankets. That's why children stay behind the legs of Dad or grab onto his pants, or thrust their heads into their Mom's neck or into her shoulders. Mom and Dad are a safe place; they trust you. What Mom and Dad tell their children, they're going to believe whether it's true or not. When you have a little three-, four-, or five-year-old come into the office to get work done, what Mom and Dad say can be a huge help to the dentist. I'll pull parents aside while one of my assistants or hygienists is talking to the child, and I'll say, "Your child has a cavity. You're going to be coming in. What I ask is just make it a positive experience. Tell them that we're going to bring the child in and we're going to be brushing one of their teeth. Just like today, it's going to be fun. Dr. Hamilton is a lot of fun, and he's going to take care of you. Get them in, get them excited, and keep them happy. Once they're in my chair, I will do the rest of the work. I will make it a good experience as long as you have my back."

It's a team effort; when a child is coming to a pediatric dentist, success comes out of a team effort between the child, the dentist, the assistant, and the parent. That's why I allow parents in the back. I have one of the few offices in which parents are welcome to come back with their child. I do that for two reasons: one, so that the parents can help us; and, two, so that they can see how wonderful we are with their kids. Many dentists do not allow parents in the treatment room with their child, and parents just go along with it. As I said before, we are in a new era in society, and in the dental field, and this is no longer acceptable to many parents.

Chapter Five

Sedation

THE WORD "SEDATION" makes some parents nervous, so let's talk a little about that. There are three different types of in-office sedation. Nitrous oxide (N2O), oral conscious sedation, and IV conscious sedation. Nitrous, of course, is the safest because it's the least invasive and performs well in reducing anxiety and producing some analgesia, or pain relief. Children with a strong gag reflex will also benefit from nitrous because it tends to suppress the gag reflex. Once you're done with the procedure, it takes approximately five minutes for the nitrous to be completely out of your system. In order to use N2O, however, the patient must be able to breathe through his nose.

There are risks attached to nitrous if the patient has certain medical problems. Nitrous on a child who has severe asthma is not recommended. Giving nitrous to a child who has glaucoma or chronic obstructive pulmonary disease is also not advisable, but it would be very unlikely to see a child with either of those complaints as they are far more typical in the elderly. If a child has sickle-cell anemia, nitrous should not be used. The last two conditions that I am aware of that would make nitrous a bad choice would be when the patient is taking bleomycin sulfate and or if the patients has a condition known as methylene tetrahydrofolate deficiency.

The most common side effects of nitrous oxide are nausea, vomiting, and headaches. The difference between nitrous in a dental setting and nitrous in a medical setting is that nitrous in a dental setting is safer because our machinery will not allow the nitrous to get above 70%. Your child will always be getting a minimum of 30% oxygen. Nitrous does a great job; it relaxes a child and allows me to talk her through the treatment process, as she's completely conscious throughout the procedure. Typically I'll use nitrous with a younger child if there's not a lot of work to be done.

ORAL SEDATION

Under what circumstances might I need to use other types of sedation? If the child is younger and there's a lot of work to be done, that's when I'll start going into oral sedation. There are two types of oral sedation that I use in my office. One is for a shorter procedure. The child is not going to be asleep, he's just going to be very "loopy," to the point where he really doesn't care what happens to him. The sedation doesn't last very long, and the time window is very short, so I wouldn't use it in a case that required extensive work to be done.

The other oral sedation medication I use is a combination of drugs that makes the child go to sleep, just as if they're sleeping at night. That allows me to do a lot more work on the child. The only time that I will not use oral sedation in the office is if it the child has a closed airway (meaning that their tonsils are really large), if they have uncontrolled asthma, if they are congested, or if they are under the age of two or under 25 pounds. In addition, sedations will not be performed on any patient who has underlying medical conditions that would pose a greater risk. I do a pre-op examination prior to the sedation in which I make sure the lungs are clear. I go over the child's complete medical history and check the vitals.

When I'm planning to do oral sedation, the child can't have anything to eat or drink six hours prior to the procedure. As a rule, we tell the parents to not let them eat or drink anything after midnight, and we make these appointments for early in the morning so the child can wake up and come straight into the dental office without having to wait at home and not eat or drink. The reason it's very important that patients don't have anything in their stomach is that sometimes medication can make the children nauseated. If they get sick, we don't want them to have anything in their stomach to vomit because then it could go back into their airway., I base the amount of oral sedation I give on your child's age and weight. All children who are under sedation are monitored for blood pressure, and pulse oximeter, which monitors the amount of oxygen in the blood supply. I use capnography, which monitors the amount of CO_2. Finally, I use a stethoscope so we can listen to the child breathing. In addition to that, I visually monitor the breathing of the child, watching the rise of the chest. My assistant is also monitoring the child. If it's IV sedation, the only thing that I add extra is the ECG monitor on their chest and another provider to monitor the patient.

FRANK TALK ABOUT THE RISKS

It's important here that we talk about the risks of these procedures as well as sedations, as I do when parents come in my office. Any time dentistry is done, there are always risks involved. Sedation only takes it to a different level. By law, these risks, as with any surgery must be disclosed. Because the patient is usually drowsy or asleep, the child may have a tendency to make a sudden movement in which case damage to adjacent structures could be involved such as the tongue, cheek, lip or other teeth. This fortunately can be addressed immediately and parents are always notified. Any time a patient is sedated, there is always a risk that the patient could stop breathing. Other risks involved are allergic reactions, infections, stroke, cardiac arrest and death. Again, by law, the risks must be disclosed. Fortunatley, I have never had any of these severe risks occur during my sedations. However, all pediatric dentists are trained in pediatric advanced life support and emergency situations. As far as I know, there has never been a report of a death of a child during a sedation in a pediatric dental office when all of the guide-lines in sedation and anesthesia are properly followed according to the AAPD. The deaths associated with conscious sedation have either been because of an overdose of local anesthetic or overdose with the drugs used. Conscious sedation is a safe and effective way to treat your children while providing a comfortable experience, as the provider is properly trained and follows the guidelines set forth by the American Association of Pediatric Dentists.

Hopefully none of this will be needed; you're actively teaching your child good oral health habits and working with them to establish good diet and hygiene, and that will show in the their oral health. But in the event that more extensive work is called for, it is both important and comforting for parents to understand what their options are.

Chapter Six

Your 6- to 12-Year-Old

FROM AGE 6 TO 12, your child's independence is increasing daily. She is spending more time on her own, with friends and at school, likely to be engaging in sports and other activities, and is increasingly making her own food choices. When children in this age range come in, I still want to talk about oral growth and development. I will take radiographs. I want to find out what the caries risk is, and I'll discuss fluoride supplements, depending on the caries risk.

I want to continue to talk about a good diet, not just with the parent but with the child as well. This age group tends to get more into sugary snacks because now they are able to reach into the cabinets and get them for themselves. By age 10 to 12, many kids are taking charge of some of their own meals as well as snacks. Now that they're more likely to be playing sports, I'll also be talking to parents and the children about injury prevention, which I'll cover a little later in this chapter.

SPROUTING PERMANENT TEETH

When your child gets those first permanent teeth at around age six, it's imperative that they begin to use fluoridated toothpaste if they aren't doing so already. Right around age six, we are getting into that mixed dentition stage, and usually, it's the lower teeth that come out first. In this mixed dentition stage, the teeth and mouth can begin to look funny because permanent teeth are coming in and baby teeth are falling out, and the difference in their size is very noticeable. You may even notice a difference in color. Primary teeth are typically whiter in color which will make the permanent teeth appear more yellow than they really are when they begin erupting. Some people call this the ugly duckling stage. Parents are concerned that teeth aren't coming in straight. This is normal. Teeth are trying to figure out how they are supposed to be coming in. Have patience, wait, and see what happens. Children are still growing, and their jaws are still growing. Even if there is slight crowding coming in, that can still be corrected with growth.

Because the lower permanent teeth erupt first, many times they'll be "lazy." They will take the path of least resistance and come in behind the lower baby teeth. If that's the case, do not panic, even though they look like shark teeth. You just need to take your child into the dentist, who can help wiggle out or extract those lower front baby teeth. The parent's concern in this situation is what effect the placement of the permanent teeth behind the baby teeth will have on those permanent teeth. The answer is that your tongue actually provides enough pressure consistently throughout the day to push those permanent teeth back into alignment where they are supposed to be.

At this age, we've discussed that kids want to brush their own teeth. Until they reach the age of 10, we encourage parents to continue to brush with them, or at least follow up until, as we said before, the child can tie his or her own shoes and they stay tied for the remainder of the day. It's imperative, too, that these children are now flossing. I start teaching parents to begin flossing with their kids once their whole primary dentition is in, which is right around age two. Now that the six-year molars are in, it's even more crucial that we floss in order to protect these permanent teeth. Cavities on baby teeth can spread over into permanent teeth, just as they can spread into other baby teeth. Unfortunately, unlike these baby teeth that will fall out eventually, these children will have these teeth—their six-year molars and the anterior teeth that come in at the same time—for the rest of their lives.

Upper Teeth	Erupt
Central incisor	7–8 yrs.
Lateral incisor	8–9 yrs.
Canine (cuspid)	11–12 yrs.
First premolar (first bicuspid)	10–11 yrs.
Second premolar (second bicuspid)	10–12 yrs.
First molar	6–7 yrs.
Second molar	12–13 yrs.
Third molar (wisdom tooth)	17–21 yrs.

Lower Teeth	Erupt
Third molar (wisdom tooth)	17–21 yrs.
Second molar	11–13 yrs.
First molar	6–7 yrs.
Second premolar (second bicuspid)	11–12 yrs.
First premolar (first bicuspid)	10–12 yrs.
Canine (cuspid)	9–10 yrs.
Lateral incisor	7–8 yrs.
Central incisor	6–7 yrs.

DEALING WITH DIET

This age group marks a point when children are spending more time away from their parents, and the parent isn't watching everything that they're eating. As is habitual in our society today, kids are snacking, snacking, snacking, and it's difficult to impossible to monitor when and on what. This is the age when they have to begin to brush their own teeth for the most part, even though they're not quite up to the task of brushing without you monitoring the job they're doing. When children come in at this age, not only do I discuss diet and diet control with parents, but I talk to the children about it too, because they're old enough to understand.

Unfortunately, even at school kids get sugary snacks. At age eight, nine, or 10, they're riding their bikes. They have their allowance. They may be running in to a 7-11 and buying candy bars or sodas. A lot of kids are drinking sodas morning to night, and the mixture between the sugar and the acid in those sodas just eats away at the teeth. It's definitely a huge concern that we talk about with parent and child.

I want to limit the sugar snacks to somewhere between one to three times a day, preferably on the lower end of frequency. When your children are thirsty, they should be drinking water, not sweet drinks. If you're going to be drinking milk and juice, limit it to snack and meal times. It's a matter of teaching your young children now and encouraging them to be partners in their own wellness because they are not always under the supervision of adults anymore. Hopefully, those habits they've learned from their parents from the earliest days are fully ingrained, and they'll start to understand their health needs and implement the right choices themselves.

FIXING PROBLEMS

Depending on the child and amount of work required, I may still do sedation with these children when they need work done. It depends on their past dental history. Hopefully, if they've been coming to see a pediatric dentist since they were young, they are trusting, and they know how things work. They are not liable to be panic-stricken or scared to come to the dentist. Actual dental work is much easier on these children. In addition, if they have been coming every six months since the age of one, I've been able to keep up with their dental hygiene, so I don't see as many caries, and the amount of work required will consequently be limited. A good pediatric dentist with an ongoing relationship of trust with their patient built up over time will usually be able to use behavior management to talk the child through the procedure.

CROSSBITES

At this stage, some kids may need appliances to correct crossbite. As I mentioned earlier, crossbite is where the teeth do not overlap in the proper manner when the teeth are together. Crossbite is often caused by the overuse of pacifiers. It's very typical to see crossbite in a child who has used a pacifier for a long time. The way that a parent can tell if a child has a crossbite is just have them close down on their normal bite. If the top teeth are not overlapping the bottom teeth—if in fact the bottom teeth actually overlap the top teeth—then the parents can see for themselves that their child has a cross-bite.

Crossbites occur both in the front and back. In an anterior crossbite. the bottom teeth are sitting in front of the top teeth.

Anterior crossbite in the mixed dentition (mixed dentition means the child has both permanent and primary teeth) is the most opportune time to correct this. The dentist will need to determine if this crossbite is of dental origin, meaning only the teeth are tipped incorrectly, or skeletal origin. If the anterior teeth are in crossbite from dental origin, and its a minor crossbite, a simple appliance can be used, which should take approximately four to six weeks to correct the problem. If its not a minor crossbite, then more agressive treatment will be warranted. If the crossbite is skeletal in origin, then you may be referred to an oral surgeon for a surgery consult.

In order to correct a posterior crossbite, it's best to treat it early on. The appliance that we use is called a rapid palatal expander, and it should be employed when children are around age 6 to 10. The reason for this timing is the process of development of the palatal shelves. The palate is not fused yet at this point, which allows the expander to correct the crossbite by actually expanding the palate. As we separate the palatal shelves a quarter of a millimeter at a time, bone will fill in the opening, which is right in the middle of the roof of the mouth. By age 12, that palate will actually fuse. Once I see that the crossbite is corrected with the palate expander, I'll let it sit there for anywhere from two to four months to let it settle before I take it out. If we take it out too early, the teeth can actually move back to where they were before.

Another reason that I want to wait until this age to recommend an appliance for a child is that this age is when their first permanent molars are in. Those molars are where I cement the bands for this appliance. This appliance is a permanent appliance. It won't come out until the dentist takes it out. The way we expand this appliance is simple. Every day, Mom or Dad will use this little tool that looks something like a screwdriver. With it, they can do what we call "activating" the appliance. Every time they activate it, this appliance will open up the palate another quarter of a millimeter. That's just one type of appliance; another type of appliance uses springs the parents don't have to activate it at all. It gradually expands on its own.

BREAKING BAD HABITS

By age six, children need to have set aside their bad habits as well; habits like thumb or finger sucking still may persist, but at this point they must be broken. If you skipped directly to this chapter, I discussed in the last chapter various ways to help break these habits. By now, your children have been practicing these habits for so long, that at night it's become second nature. The nasty-tasting and very effective finger paint, Mavala, is a great product that works like a charm. Paint it on the fingers your child prefers to suck on three to four times a day: morning, afternoon, and at bedtime. I actually used it on my own children to assist them to stop biting their nails. I painted it on my five-year-old daughter's fingers; for the next couple of days, I could not figure out why the right side of her shirt was constantly wet. Then, one day, I saw why in the rearview mirror: My daughter had forgotten, placed her fingers in her mouth, and then immediately stuck her shirt in her mouth to remove the taste. One habit to the next I guess.

Another habit that has to be corrected at this point is tongue thrusting. Tongue thrusting is where you push your tongue against the front of your mouth upon swallowing or breathing, which creates an open bite.

When all positive reinforcements fail and the Mavala isn't working, we have to move onto more stringent methods: a tongue-crib appliance. This is an appliance that is attached by two bands around your permanent molars. It looks like a little gate that sits right behind your front teeth. It keeps the fingers and thumbs from reaching the palate. The reason it's so crucial at this age to make sure that these habits are gone is because of the damage that thumb sucking, finger sucking, and tongue thrusting can do. It includes creating an open bite, which means that your upper teeth are no longer overlapping your bottom teeth. It creates a high palate, which also creates a narrow arch, where it can cause crowding. In addition, thumb and pacifier can also flare the teeth as well.

MOUTH GUARDING

Children from age 6 to 12 are getting into rigorous sports, if they haven't been already, playing tackle football, basketball, and baseball, among other things. Their teeth are at risk, and it's important to protect them, even more so now with their permanent teeth coming in. These permanent teeth are immature. The roots are not completely formed yet. I encourage all the children who are playing in any type of physical sport to use some type of sports guard. There are multiple types of sports guards out there, including some you could buy from Sports Authority, Academy, or other sporting goods stores, but the absolute best are the ones that are specifically formed for your child. That's where a dentist's office can help. I will have your child come in and I'll take an impression of his or her mouth, so that a sports guard can be made that will fit your child perfectly. With a properly fitted mouth guard, when they bite down, they're biting down correctly. A lot of the sports guards you buy at a sporting goods store are just "boil and bite." Your child is not biting down correctly and just as much damage can occur if they are hit in the mouth when they are wearing one of these guards as would happen without one. That's why a prudent parent will insist on a proper, professionally fitted sports guard. It costs a lot less than replacing lost teeth!

It's also important to note here that you don't want your child using the same sports guard from season to season. You have to be cautious because the child's teeth are changing. You want to go ahead and switch it out for a newly fitted one every year, because baby teeth are still falling out and permanent teeth are still growing in. We want to make sure these guards are continuing to fit correctly and not causing more damage than good.

You can spend a fortune on children's sports equipment. I've seen parents who will happily drop $100 on a baseball glove and $300 or more on a bat, but draw the line at buying a professionally fitted sports guard, settling instead for a cheap, do-it-yourself appliance to protect their kid's teeth, which are worth a lot more. If you were to buy a $10 sports guard that is not going to protect the teeth, you're risking not only your son's future dentition, but you may end up paying out a whole lot more than you spent on that $100 glove or that $300 bat. I've seen so many injuries in baseball, but right now, from what I see, the sport that causes the most damage to the mouths of our patients is girls' basketball. All those elbows flying around make quick work of teeth. Children in all three of your major sports—basketball, baseball, and football—

71

need to be wearing mouth guards. Hockey and lacrosse are even more dangerous to teeth. To spend $100 or $200 on a sports guard that will properly fit your child's mouth should not be seen as an "extra," but as a basic piece of safety equipment.

It's important too to know that a custom mouth guard is not just protecting the teeth, but it's also protecting the alveolus, which is the gum and bone area above the front teeth. That can mean a custom guard may help your child avoid a jaw fracture or maxillary fracture, in a situation in which a store-bought guard wouldn't give that protection.

In my exams during this stage of your child's development, I am still looking for pathology, just as I do in every other exam. I want to examine and identify any spots I see that may be out of the ordinary. If I do see a spot that looks questionable, I will perform a little biopsy. At this age, some of the things that I see that are very common are called mucoceles, which is a salivary gland that has been traumatized. Moms will see it in the lower or upper lip. It looks like a big, clear pimple that goes away and comes back, goes away and comes back. It's usually formed from trauma to the lip, or sometimes just because of the child accidentally biting the lip. We'll talk more about that in a later chapter, "Special Situations."

HORMONES AND TEETH

We've already discussed the importance of children in this age group really getting in and brushing and flossing their teeth regularly and well, and the necessity of this only increases with the onset of hormonal changes. Somewhere around the 10- to 12-year-old mark, children get into puberty. Because of their hormones, puberty gingivitis can take place, a condition very similar to pregnancy gingivitis. This is another reason it's important that these boys and girls keep up with their oral hygiene.

When the first permanent molars come in, they are larger than what your child is used to. They are formed in the body with all of these grooves and fissures, which are like little valleys and caverns on the tooth. Sometimes the child's toothbrush bristles are actually too large to get all the way down into these natural crevices on the teeth. However, bacteria are small enough to sneak down into these little grooves and fissures, and they can start forming cavities that the child can't even get to with a toothbrush. No matter what type of toothbrush it is, Oral-B, Sonicare, or a manual toothbrush, those bristles are just too large to sneak way down in those crevices. The bacteria are so tiny that they'll just sit there. Every time sugar is eaten and comes into contact with the tooth, they'll grab that sugar and start forming acid. By the time we know it, by the time we're able to see it, the cavity is already formed.

This is why, especially with permanent teeth, I do recommend what's called a sealant. A sealant is a liquid resin that I place on the tooth with a little paintbrush. The liquid resin flows down to these grooves and fissures and seals them up, so that bacteria have no place to go on the tooth. Then the toothbrush can properly clean the whole surface of the tooth. If a sealant is done properly, it's an effective preventative that works extremely well. A treatment of a sealant can last up to two to three years before it needs to be redone. It's painless, and it's completely without side effects. There's literally no downside to it, so there's really no good reason not to take this step to protect your child's teeth.

HIGH-TECH CAVITY HUNTING

Fortunately, technology for discovering cavities has improved immensely. Equipment exists that utilizes a little laser that shines over the tooth which shows whether or not the tooth has a cavity. Even if I can't see it with my naked eye, the laser will let me know if a cavity exists. Thanks to this, we can catch cavities really early, before they start spreading to other teeth or increasing in size. This is the age where children are more likely to get into gadgets and be begging you for an electric toothbrush. There's really no literature that shows that an electric toothbrush does a better job, but of course every company that manufactures them will disagree. Sonicare will say theirs is the best. Oral-B will say theirs is the best. If a manual toothbrush is used correctly, it's just as effective as any electric toothbrush.

Whatever toothbrush the child *will* use, that's the one we want him or her to have. There are toothbrushes out there put out by Disney where characters sing a song for two minutes while you brush your teeth. If your 10-year-old girl will use a brush for two whole minutes just for the pleasure of listening to Justin Bieber, that's the way you want to go. If it's a toothbrush that has a cool superhero picture on it, or if the kids love the little Sonicare or any vibration brush—whatever the children will happily and regularly use to brush their teeth is what Mom and Dad need to get. Whatever gets them excited about brushing teeth is a worthy investment.

Another advantage to these kinds of brushes is that they very often have a timer in them. It's hard for a child in this age category to realize how long two minutes is when they're in the bathroom brushing their teeth, and Mom and Dad are saying, "Hey. It's time to go to school. Get your backpack ready. Get your homework ready. Are all your papers signed? I'm going to be late for work. Get in the car." Sound familiar? Often, I'll tell the child to pick out their favorite song and brush their teeth the entire time that song is on. Most songs usually last two to three minutes.

During the years your child is six to eight, you still need to be following up; let your child do the initial brushing, then go back in and brush their teeth again. Kids who are entering the nine- or ten-year age group, are getting super independent. They don't want to have to have their mom or dad brush their teeth. What I recommend to the parents is that you give the child the opportunity to brush his or her own teeth, then let the parent take a look. I described this somewhat gross procedure earlier in the book, but the quickest and surest way to check their brushing job is for the parents to wash their hands, take their fingernail, and scrape on the front tooth. If they get any plaque off of the front tooth, then the parent brushes for them. After a while, the child will start to get the idea that, "If I brush my teeth well, then Mom and Dad won't have to follow up."

The next phase of childhood takes us into young adulthood— and a lot of new issues. We'll address your growing young person's oral health, and how it can be impacted by such lifestyle choices as substance abuse, smoking, drugs, and alcohol. We are going to be discussing new oral manifestations along with some of the common eating disorders. Kids at this age are more interested in cosmetic self-expression, so we'll talk about piercings—and whitening as well.

Chapter Seven

Your 13- to 18-Year-Old

LET'S TURN NOW to the adolescent and growing teenager. Caries incidence is actually highest during adolescence. We as dentists have done a good job of reducing caries risk in the younger population, but for some reason the incidence of caries in adolescents has stayed the same, if not increased. My guess as to why that's the case is the changing lifestyle of adolescents. At this stage of their lives, they're on their own a lot. Neither parents nor dentists will have as much control over kids in the adolescent age group as we do with younger children.

They're going to stores and restaurants on their own. They're buying their own soft drinks and candy. They may be coming in a little later at night, so parents may not be aware if they're going to bed without brushing or flossing their teeth. I'd propose that lack of oversight is why caries risk gets higher in adolescents.

TIME FOR ORTHODONTICS?

This is typically an age where all the adult teeth have erupted. Every once in a while, I'll see some primary teeth that are still hanging in there because one of their roots has not completely reabsorbed. Sometimes what happens is that the adult teeth are a little bit lazy when they're erupting, and instead of resorbing both roots, they'll only reabsorb one or only partially resorb one, which leaves one of the roots on the back teeth anchored in. If the tooth is not extracted, that baby tooth can cause the permanent tooth to shift position and to erupt in the wrong place. If it's necessary, once all of the permanent teeth are in, we'll begin phase two of orthodontics, meaning that we'll put brackets on all the teeth in order to start rotating, moving, and shifting them to where we want them to be. For a long time, orthodontics was limited only to those who had the extra money to pay, but now insurance companies will pay for some orthodontics and most orthodontics offices or pediatric dental offices will offer in-house financing; very often, the patient's credit is not even checked. We want to make it easy, so that every child out there has an opportunity to have braces.

In terms of the options available now in orthodontics for children and teenagers, you have not only the traditional braces, but you also have clear braces such as Invisalign or Simply 5. I don't know if a lot of parents are aware of those options: these brands have been around for adults for a long time, but now these companies also offer the invisible braces for teens. Braces can also be placed on the back of teeth, which hides them altogether. Ask your orthodontist about this. This is a great option for both teens and adults.

LOOKING OUT FOR TMJ

The TMJ (temporomandibular joint) is the joint in front of your ear where your jaw opens. In addition to looking at the need for orthodontics at this age, we see that TMJ problems also called TMD (temporomandibular disorder) are a very common occurrence in adolescents, both males and females. It's much more common now than it was previously, mainly because the level and intensity of physical activity has increased. These boys and girls have been playing in competitive athletics since an earlier age, and a lot of TMJ issues stem from trauma. These kinds of emerging issues are actually more commonly seen in girls than boys now, because girls are playing more sports than before. It's interesting to note too that, as females get into puberty, their hormones play a role in the TMJ issues. With the hormonal shifts we see with females, the tendons around all the joints become a little bit more flaccid, so there's more room for trauma around the joint. That's why young women are also coming down with much more frequent knee issues; the hormones affect any type of joint.

There are particular things that I look for when I'm looking at teenagers that can signal a possible TMJ problem. One is a lack of any contact between the upper and lower anterior teeth. We call that an anterior open bite. After teenagers get out of ortho treatment, if the upper anterior teeth are what we call retroclined, or tilted backward a little bit, that can be a sign that the teenager may have a TMJ problem. I also look at the degree of overbite, which means where the top teeth come over the bottom teeth; if it's zero millimeters—if there's no overbite at all—that can be a sign of TMJ related issues.

I look too for facial symmetry. If the right side of the face looks a little bit off from the left side of the face, that can lead to TMJ issues as well. I am also listening for popping or clicking. If, when you open your mouth all the way, you hear a pop or a click, you need to get in and have your TMJ examined.

The clearest way to tell you're having issues is if you're having pain in that area. If that's the case, then you need to get your TMJ evaluated, just as you would if you were having trouble with any other joint. If your knee is hurting, or if your shoulder is hurting, or your elbow, you're not going to ignore it or just monitor it, and you shouldn't take a hands-off attitude with your jaw either. If your child is having these kinds of problems, you want to get them in and get the proper diagnosis and treatment. Different imaging technologies are used to get to that diagnosis, such as MRI's. Depending on the problem, treatments for TMD can range from simply fitting the patient with a night guard, all the way to surgery and replacing the joint in the TMJ.

CONSIDERING BLEACHING

Adolescents are now coming into a new cosmetically-aware phase of life, in which they're likely to be looking at movie stars, models, and music stars as role models in terms of their ideal appearance. They want their teeth straight, and they want them to be white too, so bleaching is something they're increasingly requesting at this age.

A lot of parents I speak with are concerned about whether or not bleaching is okay at this early age because kids even as young as 12 or 13 are asking them for it. Bleaching is fine at this age but it should be done under the dentist's supervision using the most efficient and safest technology.

There are several types of bleaching methods available to you, including in-office bleaching. For in-office bleaching I'll bring the teenager in, sit him in the chair, and first put a special product over the gums to protect them from irritation. Then I'll put the bleach directly on the teeth and let it sit for 20 to 30 minutes. It makes a vast improvement just in those 20 to 30 minutes because we're working with a very high concentration of bleach in whitening those areas. We can also offer the bleaching trays to teenagers. In this method, we take a mold of their teeth, make them a special tray, and give them the bleach to take home. The parents needs to monitor this process because we've seen that if the kids are doing the bleach applications on their own, they tend to ignore the instructions given to them by the dentist and may overdo it. They have the idea that more is better, and that's not always the case.

If you're looking to try it out on your own, there are some effective over-the-counter options available too, such as Crest Whitestrips or Advanced Crest Whitestrips, which work very well. But, please—stay away from anyone without a dental license who offers bleaching. I have seen kiosks in malls, and even beauty spas offering bleaching. Many are doing teeth bleaching without the proper understanding of the chemistry behind it and the negative side effects it could have, and they do not have the capability to fix anything that they damage.

Side effects of the bleaching process may include sensitivity to gums and tissues. Sometimes, if the kids have had white composite fillings on their teeth, that white composite will not get bleached, so that tooth around the composite filling will get whiter and it will accentuate that filling. You want to be cautious of this. Also, if there are any decalcification areas on the teeth, those decalcification areas can become drastically white and show up. That typically will go away after the teeth are hydrated once again after a few days.

MISSING OR MISPLACED TEETH

When I'm doing exams on teenagers, I'm looking at malposition of teeth or sometimes even congenitally missing teeth. Malposition just means that the teeth are not in place where they're supposed to be. If we see that, we'll talk about how to move those teeth with orthodontics. Congenitally missing teeth means the tooth never developed. Some of the more common congenitally missing teeth are third molars. After third molars (wisdom teeth), the most commonly missing arethe mandibular second premolars, and after them it can be either or maxillary premolars or maxillary laterals. Hopefully, if the teen has been coming to the same dentist for several years, the dentist will have already discussed the problem with the parents and gone over the options for treatment.

Some of the options of treatment for congenitally missing teeth are to simply close the space through orthodontics or to protect that space until after the child is fully grown, which is usually around 16 for girls and around 18 or 19 for boys. Implants will then be an option. Implants are becoming the preferred, more ideal treatment, because implants replace the tooth structure in a similar fashion. Be prepared for this to be a multistage process, however, because that area might need a bone graft to help stabilize the implant.

LOOKING FOR OTHER PROBLEMS

At this stage of the game, I'll also talk to my young patients about the importance of refraining from tobacco use. The smoking habit is usually started in adolescence just through experimentation. I go into the risks of smoking and all kinds of tobacco use, including chewing tobacco and dipping snuff. I want to let these children know that major oral, dental, and systemic health problems can stem from its use. When I see patients I know are using tobacco, I do advise their parents to seek out smoking cessation programs and/or counseling. I have numbers for both counselors as well as cessation programs.

Other things we look for are oral manifestations of venereal diseases and enamel erosion. Enamel erosion can be caused by acid reflux, but occasionally, if I see enamel erosion, the first thing that comes to mind, especially if it's in a young female, is bulimia. There have been several times where I've seen the erosion, and I'll sit with the young lady and let her know that I'm here to help her out, that I trust her and she needs to trust me, and that everything that I see happening to her teeth is telling me that she is bulimic. What I find with these young ladies is that most of the time, they actually want to stop; they just don't know how. I'll ask permission to bring the parent in and usually they'll say "yes." The parent comes in and is upset, too, because most of the time they didn't know about their child's eating disorder. But now that they finally know, we have a starting point. Just realizing what this is creates an avenue to be treated.

Trauma is, again, a huge issue. As we talked about before, trauma can cause TMJ problems. It can lead to missing teeth, broken teeth, broken jaws, fractured jaws, and fracture of the alveolus, which is the bone that holds the tooth in. We can't stress enough the importance of mouth guards for all of these young men and women who are playing sports. If your child is still using an old mouth guard, get rid of it and get him or her refitted with a new one. As previously mentioned, a poorly fitted mouth guard can cause as many problems as not having one at all. We want to make sure that they have a mouth guard that is fitting their teeth correctly and covers the area above the teeth as well. Children get hit hard in a lot of games, particularly in basketball where they're not wearing any kind of other headgear that could potentially offer protection from flying elbows. Any dentist's office can make a custom mouth guard for these teenagers, because their mouth isn't changing as much anymore as they were at an earlier age. They'll be able to keep it for much longer.

ORAL HEALTH CARE

Oral health care is something I definitely want to discuss with teenagers. Unfortunately, good oral hygiene is not on the top of their list. You would think that given how important their appearance is to them, that they'd take a greater interest in it, but somehow they just don't make the connection. It's hard to get it through to a young man that, yes, his teeth do need to be white, but he also needs to be flossing and brushing every morning and night. They just hope that if bleaching gets the teeth looking good from the outside, then everything is okay. I have to educate them that, along with white teeth, they need to be brushing and flossing at the same time. Maintaining this good oral hygiene is even more important with all the hormones teens are flooded with as they're passing through puberty. Gingivitis is more prevalent at this age. Periodontitis, too, is more prevalent as you go through puberty.

Parents need to understand that even though lots of these 12- and 13-year-old boys and girls may act tough at home, sometimes the toughest-acting of them are the most terrified of the dentist. It's not unusual to get seven-, eight, and nine-year-olds who are fine with coming to the dentist, but once they hit the 11-, 12-, and 13-year-old stage, for some reason they may suddenly become phobic, or they are very anxious. The boys are a little bit easier to handle because they tend to want to look more "macho." Girls let you know right away that they are terrified. I always tell parents, "Please don't assume that coming in for dental treatment is going to be simple for them because of their age." As a parent, you need to be sensitive to this, and to make sure that you're not telling them, "Oh, yes, you're going to get shots. It's going to hurt," or even to tease your teenagers about going to the dentist's office. Despite their apparent maturity, they are just as terrified sometimes as the younger kids.

Instead, try to positively reinforce your teenager's attitude and say, "This is going to be easy. The doctor knows what he's doing. This is going to be a piece of cake. You're going to do great," rather than "It's going to hurt. You're going to get this big needle." If your teenager is experiencing anxiety, I want to do what I can to quell it, not exacerbate it. And if you yourself are fearful of going to the dentist, please do your best not to express that phobia to your children because you don't want to pass it on to them.

At this exam, I also want to evaluate the third molars. The reason you might need to extract third molars is because they're improperly positioned. Most mouths are just too small for third molars to come in properly. Third molars can lead to issues such as pericoronitis, an infection of the gum tissue surrounding a wisdom tooth. Cysts too can be an issue. Caries are very likely to occur too, because these teeth are so far back that they're difficult to keep clean. Often, teenagers or even young adults are not getting all the way back with a toothbrush to clean the third molars, so it's just better if we remove them.

I briefly touched on the topic of congenitally missing teeth. While the teen is waiting for that implant I discussed, no one wants to have a missing tooth in the front. That can cause social embarrassment that leads to big emotional disturbances and crippling self-esteem. As an example, at one of the local high schools, the captain of the cheerleading squad had an accident and knocked out her front tooth. That missing tooth made for quite an emotional issue for this beautiful girl, as you can imagine. She hadn't quite reached full growth yet, so we couldn't put an implant in—but we didn't want to leave her with that ugly gap ruining her smile. I made her what is called a Maryland bridge out of all porcelain and cemented it to the back of her front teeth. That was just temporary until we could get an implant in, but it restored her smile and her confidence in the meanwhile.

What I've discovered in working with teens is that the most important thing is getting on their level and letting them know that you are their friend. You're not just this doctor examining them and saying, "This is what you need, and this, this, and this." Teenagers, like anyone else, don't care how much you know until they know how much you care. When you walk into any office, you should have a welcoming feeling. If not, do you really want to spend your time there? Especially when we're talking about these teenagers who have some of the kinds of issues and habits that I've discussed and that do need help; if you're not their friend they're not going to trust you.

I want to talk to teens and their parents again at this visit about preventative options, like sealants on the premolar teeth, as well as on the 12-year molars. Ideally, we've already placed sealants on the six-year molars. Any time that I can do something preventative that may cost a little bit of money up front, it is important for the parents to realize that it's going to save them a lot of money and hassle in the future if they protect their kids' teeth now. In this day and age, it is no surprise to spend $500 on an iPhone and then buy a $100 protection plan for it on top of that. Then, two years later you get rid of that phone and buy a different one. Sound familiar? You might logically ask what's the difference between buying a protection plan and paying $48 per tooth for a sealant that your child is going to have for the rest of their life. You would pay $100 for a protection plan for a phone you're going to get rid of in two years. Doesn't it make better sense to pay for that sealant on a tooth that you're going to have for the rest of your life?

ORAL PIERCINGS

I see a lot of lip, nose, and tongue piercings these days on young people. They are not altogether benign; tongue piercings especially can significantly damage teeth. I see it all the time; little microfractures of upper anterior and lower anterior teeth caused by tongue rings or studs. Bacteria will sit on those tongue rings as well and will continue to stay there. I've seen people who have infections caused by the tongue ring, and obviously they can interfere with the ability to speak clearly as well.

There are even odder "fashion choices" children can make: I had an emergency situation when I was in the Air Force where a 17-year-old boy came in because he was watching the Discovery Channel and saw this guy who was trying to make himself look like a snake. He thought that was cool, and he decided he would do the same thing with his tongue—so he took a razor blade and sliced his tongue right down the middle. When he stuck his tongue out, it actually split apart. He didn't actually tell his mom what he'd done until the next morning because he was scared to tell her, and by the time she got him in to the office, some scar tissue had already formed. I had to tell the mother that in order to fix it I'd have had to actually cut the tongue in two places and sew it back up again, and she said, "No. Don't do it." He left with a little forked tongue. These kinds of impulsive acts are sort of a specialty of teenagers, who often don't think before they leap.

As doctors, we see a lot that children don't realize we can see. The effects of drug use on the mouth are very clear and easy to spot, for instance. It's these times I'll sit in with them and be very frank about it. Luckily, in the situations where I've discussed and talked to the patient, they decide they do want help. Then I actually go out and talk to the parents in the consult room by myself. I tell them very honestly, "This is what's going on. Your son is aware that I'm talking to you," or, "Your daughter's aware that I'm talking to you." I say, "This is not the time to be angry with them or mad at them. This is a time when they are asking and reaching out for help. Let's go in together. I have some numbers that you can call to get help. This is the time when we need to support them and love them." Fortunately, it's always worked out for the best.

Chapter Eight

Injuries and Emergencies

THERE ARE MANY SORTS of injuries that can occur to the facial region, but let's just cover the most common types, what to look for in assessing them, and how to treat them.

BROKEN JAW

Let's start with injuries to the face. The most common facial skeletal injury in the pediatric population is a fracture of the mandible. This occurs more often in boys than girls, but girls are starting to catch up as they're becoming more active in sports. The most common causes are from falls, bicycle accidents, car accidents, and sports-related injuries. How do you know if your child might have a jaw fracture? The first, best indicator of a jaw fracture is pain in the TMJ area. Second, if you look at their bite, you'll see that their bite will be "off," as though it's shifted to one side. Possibly, they might have an open bite, meaning the top teeth are not occluding on the bottom teeth; in other words, they're not touching the bottom teeth like they normally would. You want to look for ecchymosis, which are little blood spots or little red dots underneath the tongue. Have your child raise their tongue and if you see lots of little blood spots underneath the tongue, then that's a sign of a fractured mandible as well.

If any of these telltale signs are evident, you need to get your child to an oral surgeon right away; either call your dentist for a referral or contact a surgeon directly if you know one in your area. Treatment for a fractured mandible is usually nonsurgical. The oral surgeon will splint the upper and lower jaw together, at the proper occlusion. Sometimes they'll use some really tight elastics (rubber bands) to splint it as well. The elastic does make it difficult to eat, so purchase a good blender if you don't already have one.

If you need to stabilize the jaw while you are getting to the doctor because the child is in pain, just wrap a gauze bandage or a handkerchief under the mandible and over the top of the head and tie it off. It will help keep the chin still, keep the teeth occluded together and lessen the child's pain.

MOUTH BURNS

I talked in an earlier chapter about teething children who will sometimes bite down on electrical cords, and how that can cause terrible burns. Obviously, prevention here is worth much more than a pound of cure, and there's no substitute for properly child-proofing your home and staying vigilant.

Teething children love to bite on electric cords because they're easy to wrap their little hands around, and the cord feels good to their teeth because it's a hard plastic. If they bite through the cords—and they often will—this can cause third-degree burns, usually at the corners of the mouth. It is a terrible injury and the best thing you can do is to keep it from happening. This injury will lead to lifelong scarring, will limit the ability of the patient to open her mouth, and has an extremely painful recovery period.

INTRA-ORAL FRACTURES, CONTUSIONS

Intra-oral fractures, such as of the maxilla, occur also from blunt trauma to the mouth. Again, you want to look for ecchymosis and displacement at the maxilla (the bony area above the teeth) if you suspect a fracture. Usually you can push it gently with your finger and thumb and if you feel the bone above the tooth shifting or moving, that's an indication that there is a fracture. Look for displacement of the teeth, look for tooth mobility and if you see any of this you need to go see your pediatric dentist as soon as possible. This kind of injury will also require splinting of that fracture site for about four weeks.

The soft tissue surrounding the teeth can also be traumatized, and common injuries are contusions, which means bruising, and lacerations. Soft tissue will at times need to be x-rayed to rule out any foreign objects inside such as remnants of teeth. Depending on the size of the laceration, it may need to be sutured. The sutures are most commonly resorbable.

FRENULUM TEAR

The most common soft tissue injury usually occurs during the toddler stage, and it is what we call a frenulum tear, which is a tear in the little fold of tissue that attaches the lip to the gum. The frenulum is very fragile, and if the child falls and hits his mouth or lip, it will tear easily. It bleeds a lot, and I always warn parents that if your child should fall down and you see lots of bleeding from the mouth, don't panic. Grab a wet cloth, wipe the blood off, and assess the situation. If you see that the blood is coming from in between the gum and the lip, then it's a frenulum tear.

This is a common injury, and it will take you a good 10 minutes of putting pressure on the area to stop the bleeding, but it will eventually stop. There's no need to call 911 or take your child to the ER, and no reason to call the dentist. The area will heal on its own. The sight of all that blood can really be frightening, though, so keeping a cool head while you assess the situation is important.

ULCERS

Falls or bumps can also result in contusions of the lip, which is just bruising or swelling of the lip. An abrasion of the lip or gum tissue leaves what we call aphthous, or traumatic ulcers, which are also called canker sores. These ulcers can be very painful but typically heal within 5 to 10 days. If your child is refusing to eat and pointing to an area in her mouth, take a moment to pull the lip all the way back to check where the gums meet the lip and look for little red or white lesions. The main issue in dealing with these is keeping your child hydrated, because it's painful for them to drink.

For older kids, you can find a dentist who has a product called Debacterol. The dentist will place the Debacterol on the ulcer for three to four seconds and then rinse it off; it actually cauterizes the ulcer and then the ulcer heals from the inside and there's no more pain. Shortly, the ulcer will be gone. However, those three seconds from the Debacterol application on the ulcer before rinsing can be quite painful, so I would not recommend it for very little children.

Anything that will numb the area for a little while so a smaller child can eat is sufficient. Lasers also work well but can be pretty pricey as treatment for something that will heal on its own in a few days.

Ulcers can also be brought on by stress or caused by something as simple as eating a corn chip; the pointy end can traumatize your gum inside your mouth and cause an ulcer to happen. I see a lot of ulcers just from kids biting their cheeks, biting their tongues, and biting their lips. Ulcers are different from cold sores. Cold sores are caused from the herpes virus, not from injury or trauma.

The soft tissues of the mouth do heal amazingly fast, though. I've had parents bring their children in due to trauma and their mouth just looks horrible and in need of stitches—then a week later it looks like nothing ever happened.

TRAUMA TO TEETH

Lets discuss both permanent and primary teeth. Trauma to teeth can occur in various forms. It can come in forms of a concussion, which is a bruising of the tooth; complicated fracture; uncomplicated fracture; luxated teeth, which means displaced teeth; or avulsed teeth, which means teeth that are completely knocked out. An uncomplicated fracture means that the fracture's not into the nerve. A complicated fracture is one in which the fracture has gone all the way into the nerve. Concussion, which is bruising of the teeth, is caused when the teeth are hit, but with no further damage, meaning they weren't moved, they weren't shifted, they weren't intruded, and they weren't extruded. It's important to see your dentist for an exam, however, in order to rule out a root fracture since you can't see that kind of trauma superficially. That said, the majority of the time, these teeth do heal on their own.

Among the complications of a concussion from a tooth can be discoloration of the tooth. It can be yellow, gray, or even dark gray. The darker the color, the worse it is. In my practice, I see about 20% of those primary teeth that discolor lead to infection. At that point when the baby tooth gets infected, it will need to be extracted (or as I say in front of the child, "wiggled", so as not to scare the child).

In order to reduce the risk of that babytooth becoming infected, I recommend a procedure called a pulpectomy, which means cleaning the nerve out and placing medication to help that root area stay clean and free from bacteria. When I go in and do this, I enter in the front of the tooth, so at the same time I can put a little tooth-colored veneer on the front of the tooth so that the discoloration is gone and the tooth looks normal again. Remember, only about 20% of these teeth that are discolored do become infected, so many parents opt to do nothing and just let the tooth be, and a lot of the times the tooth just stays discolored, and it's fine until it eventually exfoliates or falls out.

Many parents will ask whether the permanent tooth was damaged. The answer depends on how the tooth was hit, and on whether the tooth was intruded on impact. The answer can also depend on how mature the permanent tooth was at the time of trauma. The risk of damage is higher if the child is under the age of three. If the permanent tooth was damaged, it would have happened right at the moment of impact. In many instances after the permanent tooth erupts, you will notice a little white spot on the front of the tooth, about the size of the tip of the root of the baby tooth. This spot is caused by the tip of the baby tooth impacting the crown of the permanent tooth. This white spot is easily repaired.

Uncomplicated fractures are fractures of the tooth that do not involve the nerve and can be fixed with only a restoration. This is the case for both baby teeth and permanent teeth. If it is a large fracture and you can find that fractured part of the permanent tooth, that can actually be cemented to the tooth without having to put a filling material on.

Complicated fractures are fractures that are large enough to involve the nerve. For primary teeth, these will need a pulpectomy or pulpotomy and usually a crown on that tooth to protect the whole tooth. On a permanent tooth, if the nerve is involved, chances are it will need a root canal. However, if it is a small exposure and you can get your child to the dentist quickly, the root canal might be avoided. Just be careful about who you choose to do the root canal, because if the root is not fully formed it may need an extra step involved to close the end of that tooth's root. It usually takes up to three years after the permanent tooth erupts for that root to be fully formed, so the extra step involved might be well worth it. Your dentist will inform you of the benefits.

Going back to the primary tooth, a pulpotomy is done on a primary tooth. A root canal is done on a permanent tooth. What is a pulpotomy? That is a procedure in which only the part of the nerve that is affected is removed. You leave all the healthy nerve in, whereas on a root canal on a permanent tooth you're removing the entire nerve.

If a baby tooth is luxated, meaning it has shifted in the mouth, you'll want to get your child to the dentist. A tooth can luxate to the side, it can luxate to the back, or it can luxate forward. You need to get to the dentist as quickly as you can because the sooner you see the dentist, the more chance the dentist has of successfully repositioning that tooth. The same goes for permanent teeth. You want to take your child to the dentist as soon as you possibly can so there will be a better chance of actually replacing that tooth in the same spot. Time is of the essence in these situations, so be prepared. Have a number handy for a pediatric dentist who is available to take emergencies, because timely treatment can make the difference between saving or losing a tooth. Chances are a permanent tooth will need to be splinted. If a baby tooth is extremely loose or is mobile, then I will need to extract that baby tooth because I don't want to risk the chance of the child aspirating that tooth.

If it's a baby tooth and the tooth has shifted but it's not mobile and it's not affecting the occlusion, I will leave it in that place. The tooth will often reposition itself. If the tooth is intruded, many times the tooth will re-erupt on its own, especially baby teeth. In permanent teeth, however, you have a much better chance of the tooth re-erupting if the root is not fully formed. Otherwise, it may need orthodontic help to re-erupt. Extruded teeth as well as luxated teeth in the primary condition may need to be extracted, depending on mobility. My biggest concern, as I said before, is the tooth falling out in the middle of the night and the child aspirating it, meaning the tooth gets inhaled. If a permanent tooth is extruded and the dentist sees the child soon enough, the tooth can be repositioned as well.

Avulsed teeth are by far the scariest of all the traumas, because that's when the tooth completely comes out of the mouth. No parents want to see their child's tooth being knocked out. If a baby tooth is knocked out, do not try to put it back, because we don't want that child to aspirate the tooth. If, however, it's a permanent tooth, here's what you need to know: again, time is of the essence. Do not try to clean the tooth. If there is visible dirt, lightly rinse with water, but do not touch or try to scrub the root or bottom half of the tooth. You need to get to the dentist within an hour of the tooth being knocked out. If you feel comfortable enough with the idea, you can try to place the tooth back into the socket yourself. To do this, hold the crown of the tooth between your thumb and finger making sure you are not putting it in backwards and with firm pressure place the tooth root first into the socket. More than likely, you will need to hold it there until you get to the dentist. By doing this, you may have saved the tooth. Most parents do not feel comfortable doing this. If not, you can store it in the child's saliva or in cold milk and get your child and the tooth to your dentist as fast as you can. With trauma, we always hope for the best, but we always want to be prepared for the worst.

Before trauma happens, do your homework: find a pediatric dentist, or contact your local hospital to find out if they have an on-call dentist. Please make sure that you have an on-call pediatric dentist and that you have his or her number programmed on your cell phone or wherever you keep your emergency numbers at home, just as you do your pediatrician's phone number. When an emergency does happen, the last thing you want to do is to have to waste precious time hunting for the help you need.

Chapter Nine

Special Medical Needs

LET ME START this chapter off by saying that of all the parents I meet, I most admire those who are parents of special medical needs children. I truly believe those parents have a gift and were chosen for their specific child. I also believe every single child on this earth is a blessing. If you're the parent of a special medical needs child, you probably are aware that those children have extra challenges when it comes to oral disease. As a caregiver, you know that oral hygiene typically is not the first priority. You're dealing with many tasks—bathing, feeding, toileting, dressing—and the need for constant supervision. Even without having any special medical needs children myself, by the time I do all that with my four kids, I'm already exhausted. I can't imagine how much more challenging it is for these folks. I don't think there's anyone more deserving of a place in heaven than those parents who care for these kids, because so much work, energy, and love must be spent on them every day.

As I stated in a previous chapter, I often tell parents of special medical needs children when they come into my office that this is one place in which these parents can have a sense of normalcy. This is one time their children can be like other children in a setting, and that setting is their dental office. A lot of times that makes the parents feel good because any other place they go, they have to alter the means by which these children are cared for, whereas at the dental office, they're the same as any other family. For me, it's a great thing.

Just like everyone else, special medical needs children must have their six-month checkup. They have to have their teeth cleaned. If there are any cavities, these cavities have to be filled. We tell these children and their parents that they have to brush in the morning and at night. They need to use floss and fluoride toothpaste. Although pediatric dentists specialize in children, nobody understands your child better than you. A wise pediatric dentist will speak to you prior to your visit in order to find out likes and dislikes, areas that help make the child calm and steps to take that will avoid extra anxiety. Prior to the child's visit, I advise the parent to meet with the dentist to discuss the dental appointment and what they can expect. I have found doing this makes for a much smoother and more enjoyable appointment for all the parties involved. I have also observed that it is best if the child sees the same doctor and assistant each time. If the practice you go to does have multiple dentists, request to have the same one.

We're only going to talk about a few of the types of special medical needs I see in my practice, including various syndromes like Down Syndrome, autism, asthma, cleft lip and cleft palate. Pediatric dentists have additional training in how to best serve their special needs patients. Any parent of a special medical needs child should certainly seek out a pediatric dentist who is trained or knowledgeable about their child's disorder.

When I see a special medical needs patient, I use a variety of behavior management techniques to gain their cooperation and get them to listen to me. Sometimes it takes a little imagination on my part; sometimes they get to hear Dr. Hamilton sing, which I promise you is no treat. They'll open their mouths usually just to get me to stop (though I do have a few fans). Some of these children don't want to get into the dental chair, so I will sit on the floor with them so that they can lie down there, and I'll do their exam with their head in my lap. There have been times where I will just leave the child in a regular office chair rather than the reclining dentist chair; they don't like the sensation of being leaned back, as it makes them feel like they're not in control. There are multiple means and variables involved in taking care of these children as they come into my office. Typically, if they do need work done, we will do it in a hospital or setting where they can be asleep and have a comfortable experience.

It's important for parents to make sure that their pediatric dentist is consulting with their physician, depending on the medical history of the child. Make sure the pediatric dentist knows the condition well enough to provide the type of treatment that is needed. Just as with any other child, we don't want these children to have a fear of the dentist, so parents need to know what oral care or oral issues are specifically related to what their child has.

Each one of these children has his or her own unique personality. In my opinion, it's the job of the pediatric dentist to find how they can relate to the children. It's not the patient that needs to adapt to the pediatric dental office; it's the pediatric dentist that must adapt to the patient. Until parents find that pediatric dentist who is willing to adjust to their child's needs, they need to keep looking.

DOWN SYNDROME

Let's talk a little bit about some of these special medical needs, beginning with Down syndrome. Down syndrome patients are some of my favorite patients in the office. Their personalities are so genuine, and they're such loving children. However, their oral manifestations can pose some issues to their oral health care. They have a larger tongue. Typically they have smaller teeth. They have congenitally missing teeth. They usually come in with an underbite. Most of them have sleep apnea. They have delayed eruption of their teeth, and they have over-retained teeth, meaning that the teeth stay in longer than is normal, so a lot of times we have to go in and extract these teeth. They have what's called dental hypoplasia, meaning that the enamel is a little bit weaker.

Generally, with Down syndrome patients, most of them won't get as many cavities, but the problem is with the gingiva. We often see that it's red, inflamed, and bleeding quite a bit. Parents definitely need to find a good, empathic pediatric dentist for their child while he is still at an early age, in order to start building that doctor/patient relationship so that the pediatric dentist can work with the family as a team in taking care of their child's oral care.

CLEFT LIP, PALATE

The structures of the face and mouth begin to take shape during the first three months of pregnancy. Cleft lip/cleft palate is the fourth most common birth defect in the US with about 1 in 700 babies that are born. Typically the parents will know right away at birth whether the child has signs of cleft lip or palate. Cleft lip and palate are among the more common birth defects, and they can range from slight to severe. One of the challenges the baby and parent face with cleft palate is feeding. Usually the infant or toddler will figure out on his own how to push the food to one side of his palate with his tongue in order to eat. If there is a struggle however, an appliance can be custom made by your pediatric dentist that is placed in the roof of the mouth in order simplify his eating. Surgeries to correct this could begin as early as seven weeks to do a surgical repair on the lip, and after that initial surgery, multiple additional surgeries will be needed. If your child has a cleft lip or palate, you want to be sure that you are involved and in the loop with the medical team dealing with the condition. This team usually consists of oral surgeons, plastic surgeons, an ENT, an orthodontist, a speech pathologist, pediatric dentist, and sometimes a counselor.

Oral hygiene for these patients can be a little tricky. Parents, do the best you can. The children with cleft lip and palate have already had so many procedures on their mouth, the last thing they want is someone getting in their mouth morning and night to brush and floss their teeth. The areas around the clefts may be more sensitive but need to be maintained as well. All of the corrected cleft lip and palate cases that I have seen have been phenomenal work by the plastic and oral surgeons. These children, boys and girls alike, will grow up having perfectly normal lives.

ASTHMA

Let's talk a little bit about asthma. Typically, most of the patients who I see with asthma are either on an inhaler or some other type of steroid. With younger patients who have asthma, if they do have multiple caries, it's very often attributable not just to lack of proper oral hygiene, but additionally because of dry mouth that's a side effect of the medications they're taking. Dry mouth, which results from decreased saliva flow due to the medications, allows the teeth to be more susceptible to cavities.

If the patient is younger, treatment can be a little riskier. Normally we don't want to sedate a patient who has uncontrolled asthma in the office. It's less risky if we take these patients to the operating room. As long as parents are maintaining the child's medications as they're supposed to be, it's not an issue. However, I do see a lot of patients come in whose parents tell me that their physician prescribed daily steroids, but once the child's asthma improved, the parents took the children off the steroids. My advice is to continue to do what the physician says, as far as the medications that are prescribed.

AUTISM

Patients with autism face many challenges when coming to the dentist. Each autistic patient has his or her own personality, and it's the responsibility of the pediatric dentist to find a way to take care of these patients. There are many autistic patients who will just not want to cooperate. You'll see in the office that the pediatric dentist often tends to be more patient than the parent is in finding a way to accommodate these kids. Whether it's singing, music, or watching

TV, the pediatric dentist has to find something in common with the patient to even get in to do an exam or treatment. The change in environment that the child encounters at the dentist office can be overwhelming.

It's important for the parents and the pediatric dentist to work together to prevent emotional trauma. Parents, do not be afraid to advise your pediatric dentist about your child's emotional and environmental preferences as well as any challenges with sensory integration such as sound, touch, texture or space, sudden movement, etc. The pediatric dentist welcomes this. Autistic children have challenges with sensory integration, and in a dental office setting, this can be difficult for the child when the dentist is wanting to be in and around their mouth. This is also new to the child, who might not understand what the dentist is trying to do. With the parent's help, a knowledgeable pediatric dentist will create a unique approach to help produce a calm environment. Many times, a child with autism prefers to be in a quieter environment, and most pediatric dental offices can offer a room with a closed door just for that reason.

The following is what you can expect at your visit. Most pediatric dentists will invite the parents back with the child. In the past, dentists might use restraint. Now, with the training pediatric dentists have, we find restraint unnecessary. Different positive behavior management techniques work well to help desensitize the child, such as "tell, show, do" or modeling. With "tell, show, do," we explain to the child what's going to happen, then show her an example, and then perform what we've described and demonstrated. For example, we tell the child we are going to count her teeth. Then we show the child how we will do it on our fingers or his fingers. We make sure to never show the children sharp-ended instruments, which tend to scare any child, not just children with autism. Then we count the teeth in her mouth. This is no different than techniques we use with other children.

Modeling may involve counting Mom's or Dad's teeth, or even the assistant's that the child is fond of, in order to show how easy it is. It is not uncommon that this takes multiple visits in order to desensitize the child to the office environment. The first visit may just be walking back to the treatment room, shaking hands with the dentist, showing some of the instruments to the child, and allowing that feeling of comfort to sink in. Remember, as a pediatric dentist, our job is to allow the child to feel important and to have a great experience, no matter the time, effort or patience that is required.

Chapter Ten

Unusual Conditions

THERE ARE SEVERAL TOPICS that I get asked about on a consistent basis that I would like to share. Let's talk a little about some unusual conditions in the mouth. Herpetic gingivostomatitis is one which we'll see anywhere from age one to age 10. Most adults have had this virus when they were young. It consists of multiple red lesions around the gums and the tongue that turns into a blister-like sores, and can be very painful. As we discussed before regarding cold sores, the treatment is just palliative, meaning that we will give a little medication to take away the pain and it will heal on its own in seven to 10 days. However, because it is so painful, children will avoid eating and drinking, which can lead to dehydration. In addition, they do not want a toothbrush in or around their mouth for the obvious reasons. So, do your best to force liquids on them and do whatever you can do to keep the teeth clean. For pain, use children's Motrin or Tylenol, and your dentist can also prescribe you a "magic mouthwash" that will help to numb the affected areas.

In an earlier chapter on injuries, we discussed what happens when a child accidentally tears the labial frenum, which is the little fold of tissue that attaches the lip to the gum. The frenum can cause spaces in between the two front teeth, and in that case it needs to be removed. You typically do not want to remove it until after the permanent canines have erupted. If the frenum has caused a gap in the teeth, we want to close the space with orthodontics before we remove it. Otherwise, scar tissue can form, and it will be very difficult to close the space between the two front teeth. These days, this procedure is commonly done using a laser that also leaves less scar tissue and allows these procedures to be performed at an earlier age without issue. It makes it very easy, causes only a minimal amount of bleeding, and typically no sutures are needed either.

Excessive lingual frenums are very common in children. Another name for this is being tongue-tied or ankyloglossia. In assessing this condition, typically we look at how far the tongue can reach over the lower front teeth. I usually do not perform a lingual frenectomy unless it's really affecting the speech (and we don't know that it's going to be affecting the speech until they're two, three, or four years old). Again, this surgery is done with a laser and typically under sedation. The laser makes for an easy procedure.

Parents come in often with concerns about when their seven-year-old child's six year molars are going to be coming in. Occasionally the molars are being blocked by the primary teeth. The good news is that 80% of the time, the six-year molars will work their way in. But 20% of the time they won't, and I will have to run interference, which sometimes involves fitting an appliance that distalizes the six-year molars. Sometimes we will need to put crowns on the second primary molar teeth, or even extract the primary molar teeth. Regardless, it's important that we allow these six-year molars to erupt.

Patients who are six, seven, and eight years old will enter the office, and I see that their four lower front teeth are extremely crowded. Mom and Dad want to know what they can do to limit the crowding. At this age, if parents do not want to place them in braces, I'll recommend extracting the lower canines. That allows the tongue to help push on the lower permanent teeth and spread the permanent teeth out into alignment. I tell the parent, this is kind of like robbing Peter to pay Paul, because we will need that space eventually. After we extract the lower canines to make room for the four permanent incisors, typically you want to put what's called a space maintainer in the mouth to hold the space. That space retainer will remain in the mouth until those permanent canines do find their way in.

Let's talk about operculums. Operculum is a big word to define a little piece of tissue that sits on top of a molar tooth. When a molar tooth starts to come in, it pushes the tissue away; the tissue has to find some place to go and usually starts to resorb backwards. Before it resorbs all the way off the tooth, the children will complain that their back teeth are hurting because when they bite down they're actually biting on this piece of tissue and it can get very tender. It can even get infected. Many times, it will heal on its own. Chlorhexidine is a liquid your pediatric dentist can prescribe that will kill the bacteria underneath this tissue and also offer some relief from pain. Then, in two to three weeks to a month, the tooth will resolve on its own. Other times, when this tissue will not resolve on its own, I want to go in and do a little minor surgical procedure to remove this tissue. It's done in the office and is very easy.

Let's talk about congenitally missing teeth. The most common congenitally missing teeth are the third molars, then the mandibular second pre-molars, then the maxillary lateral teeth, then the maxillary second pre-molars. Any time that a pediatric dentist or a dentist has to give bad news, as is the case for any doctor who has to be the bearer of bad news, it's not fun. When the dentist has to tell a parent that a tooth has to be extracted or that the child is missing a permanent tooth, it's hard on the parent. We want to make sure that we talk about what we can do to resolve the issue.

With maxillary lateral teeth congenitally missing, there are three different options. I definitely want to send these patients to an orthodontist because we either need to close the space or we need to open the space up. If we close the space, what we'll be doing is bringing the canines into the position of where the maxillary laterals were supposed to be. Once they are in the correct position, the canines can be altered to match the shape of the laterals. This is not uncommon at all and actually it looks very good. In fact, no one will be able to tell the difference unless they know what was done. The second option to replace the lateral is to put in what's called a bridge. Typically, I'll do what's called a Maryland bridge, where two little wings are attached to the tooth, and then we cement the wings onto the adjacent teeth.

The next, and probably the ideal solution in this day and age, is an implant. An implant acts as the root. The crown on the tooth will look just like the adjacent teeth. These three options are available to parents, and we'll make sure they understand them all clearly. We want the parents to be in a position to make an informed decision.

With teeth missing in the back, it's the same thing. We can create the space orthodontically and place an implant; another option is to shift all the teeth forward. Parents may say, "Well there's already a primary tooth there," when it's a second pre-molar missing and we have the baby tooth still there. As long as that baby tooth is caries-free, and there's nothing wrong with it, that is a very viable option. We can leave that baby tooth in its place. In fact, typically if the baby tooth will stay there or is there in good shape by age 20, chances are that baby tooth is going to remain there for a long time.

Besides brushing and flossing, what can I do to help prevent cavities in my children's teeth? I often get this question when a parent is doing everything they know and their child still has cavities. Other options are having your child chew xylitol gum at least two to three times a day. Xylitol is a naturally occurring sweetener that research shows reduces tooth decay. Another option to aid in reducing caries is having your dentist prescribe a supplemental fluoride gel to use in addition to your toothpaste. A third option and fairly new is a supplement called a probiotic that a child can take by mouth to kill the cavity causing bacteria.

The last two items I want to discuss briefly are mesiodens and fused teeth. A fused tooth looks like two teeth that have been pushed together. Typically both teeth have their own nerve and their own roots. It is an anomaly that occurs during the tooth's development. The tooth needs to be cleaned in the same manner. This occurs on the primary teeth and is evident in about 1% of the population. In order to tell if there are fused teeth, we count the teeth; the number of teeth will be one less than the normal count if you only count the fused tooth as one.

On occasion, a pediatric dentist will take an x-ray and see an extra tooth in the palate. It usually sits in between the two front teeth. This is called a mesiodens. It will need to be removed because it can displace your two central permanent teeth or even keep them from erupting. This is a very simple surgical procedure that can be performed in the office, and the recovery is quite easy.

We've only scratched the surface of unusual conditions, I know, but your pediatric dentist should be more than willing to discuss your child's needs with you, and happy to go the extra mile to make both you and your child feel as comfortable as possible in the office. If they're not, you may want to reconsider your choice of dentist. But do go with a pediatric dentist, and look for one who's both responsive to your concerns and proactive in finding ways to deal with your child's situation.

Chapter Eleven

Choosing the Right Dentist

IN TODAY'S WORLD finding a dentist who is right for you can be a difficult task—but finding the right dentist for your child can be almost overwhelming. With the amount of marketing and social media, you might think that any dentist will be fine or, at the other end of the spectrum, no dentist is good enough. It's definitely wise to do your homework. In this chapter, I will point out several things you should look for in your child's dentist and some "must haves."

A great way to do an initial search is via the Internet, of course. If your child is under 13, it's almost a must to seek out a pediatric dentist. You need to look at it in the same light as when you decide whether to use a pediatrician or a family physician to treat your child. You'd definitely want to take your child to see a pediatrician over a family physician while they're younger, and for the same reasons a pediatric dentist is the best choice for a young child.

Why? Pediatric dentists have at least two full years of additional training in which they are taught about the growth and development of your child from infancy to adulthood. This also includes studies in pathology that is specific to children. Pediatric dentists are also more knowledgeable in the areas of special needs and many syndromes. Pediatric dentists are trained in multiple forms of behavior management. Remember, behavior management is as necessary in working with teenagers as it is in working with toddlers. Most pediatric dentists are licensed in sedation and some in IV sedation. Pediatric dentists are usually also on staff at local children's hospitals.

Make sure when you're searching out your dentist that he or she has a website. Websites will tell you about the office, the staff, and usually will have pictures of the office and the procedures they do. That way, you can actually have the child look on the website with you so that they can get an idea of where they are going. Children do not like the unknown. They like to know what's going to happen. Many offices will now have Facebook pages as well where they will send birthday wishes or news of the office for their patients to see.

Reviews can be a great way to learn about an office, too. However, understand that there are always one or two people in this world who can never be pleased, so don't be surprised or be turned off from an office because of one or two bad reviews.

Find a pediatric dentist who is also versed in cosmetics. This way, they will be inclined to be more aware of the cosmetic and esthetic needs of their patients in addition to the functional aspects of the work they do. I hate it when I see children coming into my office with silver crowns on their front teeth. Although they're functional, it looks horrible. I would never place them on my own children's teeth, so why would I put them on someone else's? That's how a parent and a dentist need to think.

Asking your pediatrician for a reference is another way to find a dentist that you're comfortable with. Now, there are general and family dentists who have taken continuing education courses and who are good with children. Please remember, however, that it is important to create a dental home for children where they can become comfortable and learn to trust their dentist. Many family dentists are happy to see their children for cleanings and exams, but when they need treatment, they refer to a pediatric dentist. Children like to go where they feel comfortable, and it makes it more difficult for the treating dentist if they have not had time to build the relationship. If the family or the general dentist is not comfortable with the treatment, then seek out a pediatric dentist initially so the children don't have to see a new dentist or an unfamiliar face when they have that treatment done.

You may want to ask if the dental clinic has hygienists cleaning the teeth, or if it is only the dental assistants who clean teeth. In order to save having to pay a hygienist, many offices today will get their dental assistants credentialed for doing cleanings. In my opinion, it's nice to have a real hygienist cleaning your child's teeth.

Ask if the doctor uses white crowns. That includes both front and back crowns. Children can have white crowns in the back, and a lot of parents don't realize that. Many offices will only place silver. Today's age is an age of Hollywood-style esthetics, and white crowns just look more cosmetic. So many children in school already have enough issues in terms of being targets of peer cruelty. We don't need to add to that burden. Ask the doctor if he uses silver fillings, or white fillings, because that can have a real impact on the child's appearance too.

Find out what the office's dental mission is. Is their primary care goal the care of kids? Or do they also treat adults? If so, you should ask yourself which you would rather have: an office that is focused entirely on children, or one that is not. Are the doctors active in their associations, such as the ADA (the American Dental Association) or AAPD (American Academy of Pediatric Dentistry)?

You want to ask or find out what technology the dentists have in their office. Did you know that there are bitewing x-rays that can be taken on children for which nothing has to be placed in the child's mouth? Those old bitewings that hurt your mouth or were hard to close on are not the only option any longer. We have an x-ray unit that just goes around the child's mouth. It takes bitewings, so it makes it very easy and convenient for the child.

Did you know there is fluoride that can be placed so that your child does not have to wait 30 minutes to eat or drink? They can eat or drink almost immediately. Did you know that there are techniques where the shots given can be almost painless, if not truly painless? In fact many of my patients are laughing when I give them their injection or shot.

Make sure the dentist you choose is using digital x-rays. The dosage of radiation patients get is so minimal nowadays, thanks to these digital x-rays. You get as much radiation rowing a boat for five minutes in the sun as you do from taking bitewings in a digital dental office.

Ask what the typical wait time is in the waiting room. For example, if the appointment is at 2:00, you need to be seen at 2:00. There's nothing more frustrating than showing up to your dental appointment and having to wait 25 to 30 minutes to be seen. This goes back to how well the office is run, and that matters to me and to my patients. My staff knows that no one is to wait longer than 10 minutes in the waiting room.

Does the dentist offer paperless service? Are they offering convenient online forms where you can actually fill out all the paperwork there? They should be. That way, when you get into the office they already have it, and your child can go right back to get their cleaning or their exam.

Customer service is huge. In this day and age, no one should accept less than perfect customer service. Disney is what I've always used as the great example. I train my staff to take after Disney. From the moment someone enters the door and before they have even come two steps in, they must be greeted. None of my offices have closed windows at the counter. They're all open. I don't ever want a patient to feel shut off. You know what I'm talking about, right? When you walk in and there's a glass door that the front office has to slide open to greet you? None of my offices have that sliding door. It's all an open field so that the patient is just as much a part of the dental clinic as we are.

My team knows they're to greet the patient by name. If they don't know the patient's name, they need to shake hands and introduce themselves. It is important for the children and parents to feel welcome. Before my offices open, everyone knows to put on their Disney face. Going back to when they're shaking the parent's hand, they also get down on the level of the child, down on one knee, and greet the child eye to eye and by name. Every moment of your experience should be optimal, welcoming, and warm. We say that if Disneyland is the happiest place on earth, then iKids is a close second.

Find a dentist who smiles. That shows that he or she is happy and wants to be there with your child. There's nothing more discouraging than to walk in and the dentist or the treating doctor is not happy.

Does the dentist you're considering offer emergency services after hours? Too many times teeth are lost because parents cannot find a dentist willing to come in at 10:00 at night, so they end up in the ER waiting an hour or two only to hear a physician tell them to see their dentist the next day. Mouth injuries are time sensitive. The sooner you seek treatment, the better off your child will be.

Does the doctor or the dentist that you're considering allow parents in the treatment room and in the back? So many children are timid. They do feel more comfortable when their parents are around. Now, it's important to let the doctor do his job while you're back there, and not to interfere of course, but I have been letting parents come back to the treatment rooms from the very beginning. It just makes for a much more enjoyable experience and visit for both the parent and the child. On the other hand, if the child does want to come back alone, by all means, let him feel that sense of accomplishment and parents can enjoy a moment of peace in the waiting room. At least find an office that gives a parent the choice.

Finding the right dentist is an important step in your child's life, and one to which you should give due consideration. The first visit to the dentist should be by their first birthday.

I hope this book has helped answer your questions about your child's oral health and development. My door is always open if you have any I didn't cover.

TOOTH ERUPTION CHART

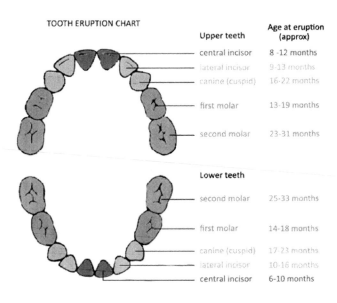

Upper teeth	Age at eruption (approx)
central incisor	8 -12 months
lateral incisor	9-13 months
canine (cuspid)	16-22 months
first molar	13-19 months
second molar	23-31 months

Lower teeth	
second molar	25-33 months
first molar	14-18 months
canine (cuspid)	17-23 months
lateral incisor	10-16 months
central incisor	6-10 months

Upper Teeth	Erupt
Central incisor	7-8 yrs.
Lateral incisor	8-9 yrs.
Canine (cuspid)	11-12 yrs.
First premolar (first bicuspid)	10-11 yrs.
Second premolar (second bicuspid)	10-12 yrs.
First molar	6-7 yrs.
Second molar	12-13 yrs.
Third molar (wisdom tooth)	17-21 yrs.

Lower Teeth	Erupt
Third molar (wisdom tooth)	17-21 yrs.
Second molar	11-13 yrs.
First molar	6-7 yrs.
Second premolar (second bicuspid)	11-12 yrs.
First premolar (first bicuspid)	10-12 yrs.
Canine (cuspid)	9-10 yrs.
Lateral incisor	7-8 yrs.
Central incisor	6-7 yrs.

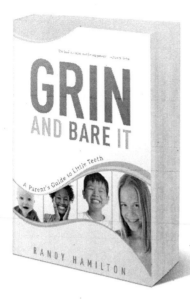

How can you use this book?

MOTIVATE

EDUCATE

THANK

INSPIRE

PROMOTE

CONNECT

Why have a custom version of *Grin and Bare It?*

- Build personal bonds with customers, prospects, employees, donors, and key constituencies

- Develop a long-lasting reminder of your event, milestone, or celebration

- Provide a keepsake that inspires change in behavior and change in lives

- Deliver the ultimate "thank you" gift that remains on coffee tables and bookshelves

- Generate the "wow" factor

Books are thoughtful gifts that provide a genuine sentiment that other promotional items cannot express. They promote employee discussions and interaction, reinforce an event's meaning or location, and they make a lasting impression. Use your book to say "Thank You" and show people that you care.

CPSIA information can be obtained at www.ICGtesting.com
Printed in the USA
BVOW05s1117240414

351606BV00013B/355/P